29.95

D0571658

# Dr. David Reuben's

# Quick

# Weight-Gain

# Program™

OTHER WORKS BY DR. DAVID REUBEN

*David Reuben's Mental First Aid Manual: Instant Relief
from 25 of Life's Worst Problems*

*Everything You Always Wanted to Know About Nutrition*

*The Save-Your-Life Diet Cookbook*

*The Save-Your-Life Diet*

*To Get More Out of Sex*

*Any Woman Can!*

*Everything You Always Wanted to Know About Sex*

# Dr. David Reuben's

# Quick

# Weight-Gain

# Program™

## David Reuben, M.D.

Crown Publishers, Inc.
New York

**T**o my darling wife, Barbara,
who made this book possible—as
she makes *Everything* possible . . .

APR 1 1 1996

*The words "Quick Weight-Gain Program" constitute a valid trademark and cannot be used without the permission of the trademark owner.*

Copyright © 1996 by Lagora Investments, Inc.

Published by Crown Publishers, Inc., 201 East 50th Street, New York, New York 10022.

CROWN is a trademark of Crown Publishers, Inc.
Manufactured in the United States of America
Library of Congress Cataloging-in-Publication Data
Reuben, David R.
    [Quick weight-gain program]
    Dr. David Reuben's Quick weight-gain program / by David Reuben.—
1st ed.
        p.    cm.
    Includes index.
    1. Leanness—Prevention.  2. Leanness—Diet therapy.   I. Title.
RA784.R48  1996
613.2′4—dc20                                              95-30354
                                                              CIP

ISBN: 0-517-70205-3

10  9  8  7  6  5  4  3  2  1

First Edition

# Contents

# Acknowledgments

I would like to thank Ben Camardi, of the Harold Matson Co., my agent, for his loyalty and tenacity. I would like to thank my editor, Jane Cavolina, for her help from the first word of this book—and even before that.

I would also like to thank my wife and children—the results of their love and dedication appears on every page.

# Introduction

## Underweight Is a Killer Disease

It has been said that a woman can never be too thin or too rich. As a witty remark it's fine. As medical advice, it's in far left field. In the headlong rush to imitate the emaciated young ladies and gentlemen in the fashion magazines everyone seems to have forgotten that up to 48 million[1] underweight Americans struggle every day to keep from getting even thinner. That's right—48 million underweight Americans—calculated according to the strict "Dietary Guidelines for Americans" of the U.S. Department of Agriculture, as well as the criteria of the National Academy of Sciences, the National Center for Health Statistics, the Canadian Ministry of National Health, and the World Health Organization. It's one thing to step on the scales in the morning and see that you've put on a pound or two. That's annoying. But imagine how it feels to lose more and more of your already scanty fat, muscle, and connective tissue as each day goes by. It's your precious body that's disappearing bit by bit in spite of all you can do to eat as much and as often as you can.

No one whose weight is normal—and much less someone who is overweight—can really appreciate the frustration of being thin—and getting thinner. And the wonders of Space Age Medicine aren't much help. Listen to what one of my underweight and unhappy patients remarked to me only yesterday. Her name is Helen, she is 27 years old, 5 feet 3 inches tall and weighs 91 pounds.

"I went to my family doctor and told him I was too thin and I wanted desperately to gain weight. He laughed and said, 'Come back after you have your first baby and I'll help you *lose* weight. I don't have time to treat imaginary problems.' ''

But underweight is not an imaginary problem. In some strange lapse Medical Science seems to have developed collective amnesia as far as underweight is concerned. Not too many years ago—as recently as the 1940s—medical texts and medical journals were replete with articles dedicated to the serious problems of underweight. Then, little by little, victims of underweight were shoved into the background as the very profitable business of "weight reduction" grew and prospered. Fast food and a slow life style made millions of people puffy while the chronically thin got even thinner—and even more forgotten. I know what plump people say: "I'd give anything if only I had that problem! Why should anyone complain about being underweight?''

Just for the record, here's why.

1. Underweight can be fatal. Up to 5 percent of all the deaths in the United States are attributable to underweight.[2] That adds up to 120,000 deaths per year, making underweight the fourth most frequent cause of death in the United States[3]—after death by strokes and more common than accidental death.

2. In a recent medical study of 608 underweight women[4] (their subnormal weight was confirmed by a reliable scientific measurement known as the "BMI") [or Body Mass Index] more than one-third suffered from significant menstrual problems, chronic fatigue, neck pain, and stomach problems. These problems are everyday experiences for millions of underweight American women.

3. There is now conclusive scientific evidence that people who are underweight have a much greater chance of dying prematurely than those whose weight is normal.[5] Underweight is a serious medical problem.

4. For years pregnant women were exhorted to keep their weight

down—at all costs. But now we know that pregnant women who are even moderately underweight have a much higher rate of anemia, frequently have undersized, apathetic babies,[6] and more of their babies die around the time of birth.[7]

If we take all these facts into consideration it becomes obvious that underweight is one of the most serious medical problems in America today. That's the bad news. But the good news is this: Underweight can be cured successfully—without drugs, without expensive treatments, without risk to the patient. All it takes is a profound awareness of the problem, an understanding of the simplest and most successful methods of treatment, and the dedication to help every person who is underweight regain their normal weight.

That's exactly what Dr. David Reuben's Quick Weight-Gain Program™ offers you. To get started, just turn the page . . .

# An Open Letter to My Fellow Physicians

Dr. David Reuben, M.D.
The Harold Matson Co.
276 Fifth Avenue
New York, N.Y. 10001
Tel: 212-679-4490
Fax: 212-545-1224

Dear Colleagues:

It has been a while since I had the pleasure of addressing you collectively. As you will remember, the last occasion was in the introduction to my book *The Save-Your-Life Diet,* where I introduced the high-fiber diet to America.

Now I am happy to present a new book which in its way is just as exciting. Just like you, I was brought up in the era of "weight-phobia." We were taught—in medical school, in internship and residency, in post-graduate courses, that our patients' greatest enemy was overweight. You and I treated thousands of sick overweight people and we understood the problem. But there was another problem—just as important—that no one ever told us about and is just as dangerous, if not more so. I came across it quite by accident a year or so ago in my ongoing research in the world of medicine. That problem—tragically overlooked yet potentially lethal—is underweight.

And it's not a small problem. I believe you will be as shocked as I was to learn that according to the Guidelines of such prestigious groups as the U.S. Department of Agriculture, the National Academy of Sciences, the National Center for Health Statistics, the Canadian Minister of National Health, and the World Health Organization, as many as 48 million Americans are presently underweight. Furthermore, up to 5 percent of all the deaths in the United States are attributable to underweight.[1] That adds up to 120,000 deaths per year, making underweight the fourth most frequent cause of death in the United States—after death by strokes and more common than accidental death.[2]

The purpose of my latest book, *Dr. David Reuben's Quick Weight-Gain Program,* is to help patients understand the real dangers of underweight and to encourage them to cooperate with you in their treatment. I hope my book will be helpful in explaining to your patients some of the complex aspects of dealing with underweight. In that way, you will have more time in your busy schedule to devote to the actual treatment.

If you have any questions, if you would like a copy of a concise bibliography, or if you would simply like more information, please feel free to contact me by letter, fax, or telephone. You can be sure of a prompt and personal reply.

With warmest wishes for your continued success and good health,


Fraternally yours,

*Dr. David Reuben, M.D.*

Dr. David Reuben, M.D.
DR/ath

## To My Readers

**D**o not attempt a weight-gaining program unless and until you have had a thorough examination and consultation with your physician. As with any diet program, if at any time during the program you experience any discomfort or serious symptoms consult your physician immediately. If you experience any pain or discomfort during any of the recommended exercises stop immediately and consult your physician.

## The United States Food and Drug Administration

**T**he Code of Federal Regulations of the United States Food and Drug Administration, Title 21, Chapter 1, Section 3, 41, page 90, says:

It is therefore the opinion of the Food and Drug Administration that any claim, direct or implied, in the labeling of fats and oils or other fatty substances offered to the general public that they will prevent, mitigate, or cure diseases of the heart or arteries is false or misleading, and constitutes misbranding within the meaning of the Federal Food, Drug, and Cosmetic Act.

## Chapter One

# The New Way to Tell If You're Underweight

The first step in our program to gain weight is to ask the critical question:

"How do I tell if I'm underweight?" There are some simple and reliable ways to tell and as we go along we'll explain exactly how to use them.

But first of all, don't worry—if you're underweight you have plenty of company. It may come as a surprise but up to 17 percent of American men, women, and children are below their healthy and desirable weight. According to authoritative medical surveys, as many as 48 million Americans are underweight. As a direct result of being underweight, you run a real risk of serious illness, a substandard quality of life, and worst of all—dying well before your time. Underweight is much more than just being "skinny"—it is a condition that undermines your health and your well-being.[1]

And it can ruin your children's life as well. Women who are underweight run a real risk of giving birth to undersized, unhealthy, apathetic babies, and all too many of their babies *die* before, during, or after birth.[2]

But that's only the tip of the iceberg. Underweight people suffer financially too. Many important and attractive job opportunities are off limits to them. Police officers, firefighters, and security guards—among others—have to meet minimum weight standards. So no matter how capable, how experienced, and how motivated a person may be, underweight slams the door of opportunity in their face. More subtly but just as tragic, in the hundreds of thousands of jobs that require a public "image," underweight folks get the "don't call us, we'll call you" routine. That includes everything from receptionists and hostesses to lucrative sales jobs and the bulk of positions in the area of "public contact" and "public relations."

And if the health hazards and the financial loss aren't enough, the emotional suffering can be intense. Like it or not, we live in a world of expectations. Women are expected to have full rounded hips, clearly delineated breasts, full calves, and attractive legs. Men are expected to have broad shoulders, well-developed arms and legs, and a "weighty" presence. Men tend to choose women who fulfill these "expectations" and women tend to choose men the same way. It's not fair; but unfortunately that's the way it is. And often the reactions of the outside world are cruel and painful. Charlene's case was typical.

After months of indecision as summer approached, she finally did something few underweight women dare. She bought a two-piece bathing suit. Reasonably satisfied with the way she looked, on the first warm day she ventured onto the beach. After a few minutes of basking in the sun, she decided to take a dip in the ocean. As she arose from her beach blanket and took the first step toward the water she heard the woman behind her remark loudly to her husband,

"Oh, look at that awfully scrawny woman! Why, she's just skin and bones!"

That took all the fun out of Charlene's day at the beach and cast a shadow over her entire summer.

For underweight folks, every trip to buy clothes can be an ordeal. Underweight women often haunt the girls' department for their outfits—and sometimes they have to even turn to boys' clothing stores to find the sizes they need. And of course, the clothes don't really fit. A girl is not a woman and a boy even less so. Beyond that, the styles just aren't the same. That's what bothers Marilyn:

"You know, Doctor, I'm a receptionist at a major medical clinic. I'm 25 years old, 5 feet 3, and I weigh one hundred and three pounds.

I haunt the girls' department and the boys' department at the clothing stores and most of the time I find clothes that I can barely get by with. But it's not the 'medical clinic look' exactly. You know what the styles for kids are like! Sometimes the doctors arrive in the morning and ask me things like, 'How was the rock concert?' or 'What band do you play in?'

"It's embarrassing and one of these days it can cost me my job. And when I go out on a date? Somehow they don't stock a nice sexy basic black dress in the 'contemporary teens' department."

And it's not much easier for men. Listen to what Roger says:

"Sometimes, Doctor, I feel like I live in a different world—as if nobody knows I'm here!"

"What do you mean, Roger?"

"Well, take clothes for instance. I'm 5 feet 11 and I weigh 133. I'm an account executive with a major advertising agency and I have to call on our clients. I have three or four meetings every day. I'm talking to presidents of big companies—you know these fellows are sharp dressers. And here I am with a shirt collar that gapes around my neck. If I get a shirt with a collar that fits, it's a size so small that the sleeves are halfway up to my elbows. If my suit jacket fits in the shoulders, there's enough room to shoplift a television set between me and the front button. Even if I buy the top brands, I end up looking like I did my shopping in the Salvation Army store in Beverly Hills! It's all name brands but sized for three different people!"

"Have you found a solution?"

Roger smiled grimly.

"Sure. I have my suits and slacks and shirts custom-made. In my business, appearance is everything and I have to make a good impression. A simple suit costs me about $850 and I can get a plain white shirt for about $98 if I buy three at a time. Slacks are only $190 and fortunately I don't need custom-made underwear. I use safety pins to tighten up my shorts because no one sees it. It's not exactly the way I want to do it, but until I put on some weight, I don't have much choice.''

When it comes to personal relationships, things aren't much better. Beth's experience is typical.

''You know people have said that our culture has a breast-fixation. Well, I'm not in any danger of that because before you can have a breast-fixation, you have to have breasts. Would you believe a 31½ A cup? It's like the old joke—I thought I was putting my bra on backwards until I realized I was putting it on the right way? Only it's no joke.''

Beth shrugged.

''It's not that I want to become a sex symbol exactly but I want people to know whether I'm coming or going. Well, I guess you can tell by all the jokes I make about it that it really bothers me. I mean, I can't wear a decent sweater, I don't fill out my blouses and I can't even imagine going to the beach. I know what the problem is—I weigh 102 and I'm 5 feet 5. I know that breasts are mostly fat and I just don't have any. And speaking of fat, I can't sit on a wooden chair. I don't have any padding anywhere on my body—it's like I don't have a rump. You can imagine how I look in tight jeans.''

She shook her head.

''But it's not really the clothes or the chairs that bother me. Men just don't go for a girl who doesn't look like a girl. No breasts, no derriere, no curves—and I like men, I like romance, I like to feel sexy—but I just can't get started.''

Fortunately for Beth, the *Quick Weight-Gain Program* solves all those problems. There are even special techniques that make sure the breasts and hips get their share of development as the pounds go on. (You'll read about them in detail in chapter 5.) Before Beth's diet program is over, she'll be able to wear sweaters, sit on wooden chairs, and stroll proudly around the beach like anyone else.

The truth is, for those who are underweight, adding pounds opens the door to a better life in every way. As you gain weight, you gain better health, longer life, better job opportunities, and better personal relationships. In a real sense, when you gain weight, you gain everything else.

But how do you know if you are really underweight? There are several answers to that question—depending on what your goals are. In general, if you *think* you are underweight, you *are* underweight. If you look in the mirror and see scrawny arms, spindly legs, a thin neck, and sunken cheeks, you are underweight. If you are a woman and you have a flat chest, straight hips, and thin buttocks, you are underweight. If you can't sit comfortably because you don't have enough padding, if your clothes hang on you instead of fitting you, you are underweight.

Of course everyone has the freedom to decide if they *want* to be underweight. Some people like the idea of being thin, bony, and angular. But most of us prefer to reach a well-rounded normal weight. Most of us like to be attractive aesthetically and sexually. Most of us like the added protection against unforeseen illness or accident that a normal weight reserve gives us.

As we said, anyone who feels they are underweight can follow the *Quick Weight-Gain Program* and easily and safely add those missing pounds. To make it even easier and more efficient, it helps if you have some scientific measurement of really how underweight you are and how close you are getting to your goal of normal weight. Unfortunately for the past hundred years or so it wasn't that easy. All we had to go by was the famous "height and weight tables." They used to be on the front of the penny scales and in the back of "Family Medical Encyclopedias"—and in the high school gym coach's desk drawer.

But these tables had a few defects that were obvious to everyone. All human beings are different—some of us have big bones and big frames, some of us have little bones and small frames. And some of us have thick heavy bones and small frames.

The weight tables tried to deal with that problem by specifying three or so kinds of "frame" or stature for each weight category and dividing the ideal weights into separate groups for men and women. It was better than nothing but it was far from ideal. The tables were also criticized by experts for not accurately representing the weight status of all the different ethnic groups in the country, for their limited number of "frame sizes," and for being based on entire populations instead of individual people.

What we doctors really needed was a way to calculate the ideal weight for each person individually—automatically taking into account the infinite variations in frame and bone size and other obvious differences between one person and another.[3] Fortunately, several years ago, that problem was solved.

There is a new and brilliant weight-tracking system that works equally well for men and women of all sizes and shapes. It is so perfect that it is used as an official standard by the U.S. Department of Health and Human Services, the U.S. Department of Agriculture, the National Academy of Sciences, the National Center for Health Statistics, the Canadian Ministry of National Health and Welfare, and the World Health Organization.

This ideal system is called the "Body Mass Index," or "BMI" for short. By using this method, you can quickly calculate exactly how much underweight you are. Just as important, as you add pounds with the *Quick Weight-Gain Program* you can measure your progress accurately. The calculations are extremely simple once you go through it the first time. *But you'll never have to do it!* It's calculated for you in the special tables farther along. But you might be interested to see how the calculations are made—it helps to understand how useful the BMI is.

All you need is two numbers. The first number is unique for everyone and *never* changes unless you gain or lose height. (Yes, with age people tend to lose height.) We can call it your "frame number." It represents the kind of frame you have and instead of "small," "large," and "medium," it covers the thousands of subtle differences that make you unique and different from everyone else in this world.

The second number is simply your weight—expressed in kilograms instead of pounds. That will change as you gain weight. So to instantly calculate your progress all you have to do is divide your weight—which changes—by your frame number, which *never* changes unless you are growing taller or shorter. The calculations are super-simple—you won't have to spend much time on them— don't be afraid. And to make it even easier, you *don't* have to do the arithmetic yourself. You can find your BMI *automatically* by using the tables in the appendix. But if you're curious about how we figure the BMI, here's an *example* of how it works:

### To Get Your Frame Number

1. Take your height in inches.
2. Multiply it by 2.54 (a pocket calculator is a big help at this stage).
3. Divide that number by 100.
4. Multiply that number by itself.

That's it!

To show how easy it really is, let's figure Marilyn's frame number. She is 5 feet 3 inches tall:

1. Height in inches: five feet times 12 inches to a foot = 60 inches. Plus three inches since she is five feet three inches tall. So, her height in inches is: 63.
2. Multiply by 2.54 = 160.
3. Divide by 100 = 1.6.
4. Multiply that number by itself. $1.6 \times 1.6 = 2.56$.

That's Marilyn's frame number. And as long as she doesn't grow (or shrink), it *never* changes.

Now let's calculate her weight in kilograms. All we have to do is divide her weight in pounds by 2.2. (The calculator comes in handy here as well.)

**1.** Weight in pounds = 103
**2.** Divide by 2.2: 103/2.2 = 46.8

That's it!

Now let's see what Marilyn's BMI turns out to be. Her weight in kilograms, 46.8, divided by her frame number, 2.56, gives a BMI of 18.28.

How does that stack up? Well, let's check it against the U.S. Department of Agriculture and the U.S. Department of Health and Human Services guidelines for ideal weight. The normal BMI range for men and women between 19 and 34 years old is from 19 to 25 kilograms per square meter. (That's the good part of the BMI—it measures weight per square meter so it accurately reflects the percentage of body fat.) Marilyn at 18.28 is definitely underweight. The next question is just as important: How much should Marilyn weigh?

That's an easy calculation. Assume that she wants a middle-of-the-road BMI at, say, 22.5. All she has to do is multiply her frame number, 2.56, by her ideal BMI, 22.5 in this case. That gives her 57.6, which is her ideal weight in kilograms. Then multiply by 2.2 to give her ideal weight in pounds: 126.72, say 127 pounds. Since she weighs 103 pounds now, she has to put on 24 pounds to reach her ideal weight—an easy job for the *Quick Weight-Gain Program.* (But remember you don't have to do these calculations—almost all the work is done for you in the appendix.

Be sure to write down your current BMI and your ideal BMI just so you have a record.

| Date | Current Wt. | Current BMI | Ideal Wt. | Ideal BMI |
|------|-------------|-------------|-----------|-----------|
| 10/24/96 | 103 lbs. | 18.28 | 127 lbs. | 22.5 |

Those five numbers are all we need to get started on our fast and easy weight-gain program—at a single glance they tell us all we need to know. We have the date we started, how much we weigh, and how much we want to weigh. But most important of all, we have our Body Mass Index that tells us precisely what our progress is and how valuable it is to us. There's only one more step to take before we can get down to the exciting details of putting on those pounds that we need so much.

If we have lost weight lately or just haven't been able to gain the way we would like, the most likely explanation is simply we're not eating right, not following a scientifically sound weight-gain plan, and not doing the things we need to do to keep our weight up there where we want it. As a matter of fact, up to 71 percent of people who lose weight without wanting to have no serious physical illness whatsoever. But just to be on the safe side, before starting the *Quick Weight-Gain Program*—or any other diet—it always makes sense to pay a visit to your doctor. It doesn't make sense to try to gain weight if there is some underlying physical cause behind your underweight. The first step is to clear that up—if possible—and then forge ahead in your weight-gain program.

There are some tests that have proven very useful over the years in checking people who are about to embark on a weight-gaining program. Here's the list—along with a brief explanation:

1. Complete Blood Count (CBC). This counts the number of red blood cells and white blood cells and checks out their size and shape. It detects anemia, leukemia, certain infections, and other problems.
2. Sedimentation Rate (ESR). This measures how fast the components of your blood settle out. It detects infections and other problems.
3. Urinalysis. Excellent for identifying kidney and bladder problems.
4. Chemistry Multiphasic Panel (CMP). This is a combination of strategic tests that pinpoint any serious conditions. It usually includes tests for kidney function, liver enzymes, albumin, calcium, and phosphorus. It also measures various chemicals in the blood and—very important—checks blood sugar to detect diabetes.
5. Chest X-Ray. Important to detect tuberculosis or lung tumors.

**6.** AIDS test, if appropriate: To put it mildly, AIDS can keep you from gaining weight.

There are five other special tests for special cases—your doctor won't overlook them but you may want to remind him. They are:

**I.** Test for blood in stool (if over 40 years old). In the earliest stages of cancer of the colon there are hardly any serious symptoms *except* for the appearance of tiny invisible amounts of blood in the bowel movement. Your doctor can detect that blood by a simple, inexpensive, but very sensitive, test.
**2.** Sigmoidoscopy [flexible type] (if over 50 years old). This test involves examining the colon by inserting a thin flexible tube through the rectum and looking for tumors or polyps. (A polyp is a kind of tumor or swelling on the end of a short stalk.) It's not a difficult test and worthwhile to detect any potential problems.
**3.** Pap smear in women. This consists of examining cells wiped off the surface of the cervix under a microscope. It detects cancer of the cervix simply and easily.
**4.** Mammography in women (if over 50 years old). This is a relatively new technique of detecting breast cancer by X-raying each breast.
**5.** Prostate-Specific Antigen in men (if over 50 years old). This is a simple blood test that detects a chemical in the blood associated with cancer of the prostate gland.

Of course there is a very small possibility that you have any of these diseases but it's better to eliminate that possibility at the start rather than struggle unsuccessfully to put on weight and wonder why you don't make any progress.

There's one other area we have to cover. It's a story that goes back to 1935. Back then a strange and mysterious businessman suddenly appeared on the American scene offering a guaranteed treatment for overweight. All the patient had to do was take one

THE NEW WAY TO TELL IF YOU'RE UNDERWEIGHT · 11

single capsule and a slim and fashionable figure was guaranteed for life! To make it even more exciting the patients were allowed to eat as much as they liked—with no restrictions. They could eat ice cream, fried foods, milk shakes, pizza, cheeseburgers, and anything else. It didn't matter—permanent weight loss was guaranteed!

You can imagine how many capsules that promoter sold. And the amazing thing was that it worked! The customers—mostly women—began losing weight a month or so after taking the capsule even if they ate constantly. It was like a dream come true. They could eat immense lunches and gigantic dinners and snack in between meals. It didn't matter. They retained a slim and fashionable figure. They were delighted! But (and I'm sure you realized right from the start that there had to be a big "but") the weight loss continued month after month. They became thinner and paler as each month went by. It wasn't long before they all became so weak they could hardly stand. When they finally showed up by the hundreds in their doctors' offices, the diagnosis was clear.

Each and every one of the "weight-loss" capsules contained a hefty dose of hookworm eggs! The unsuspecting women took the capsules, the eggs hatched, and the hookworms grew inside their intestines and thrived by sucking their blood. No matter how much they ate, the hookworms ate more and gradually they became thinner and thinner and weaker and weaker.

What does that mean to us on a weight-gain program? Just this. A few decades ago we wouldn't even have to think about intestinal parasites. But the world has become a lot more contaminated than ever before. With the increased mobility of millions of people, there are intestinal parasites now where we least expect to find them. Unfortunately as many as 25 percent (or more) of all Americans have intestinal parasites at any given moment. And one of the greatest enemies of success in a weight-gain program are those thousands upon thousands of invisible worms and other parasites that can make their home in your intestines. If you are infested with parasites, you can eat ravenously, you can struggle and struggle to gain weight and still you won't make any progress. The thousands and thousands of tiny monsters that occupy your body against your will suck the nutrition out of everything you eat. Be sure to have your doctor test you for intestinal parasites before you start. The medical term for the test you want is "Stool for Parasites and Ova." That means the doctor checks a small sample of your stool for adult intestinal parasites as well as their eggs that will soon hatch. Obviously hookworms are among the most dangerous common intestinal parasites but make sure your doctor checks you for other creepy-crawlies like amoebas, whipworms, roundworms, tapeworms, and Giardia Lamblia.

If you have traveled to exotic tropical places be especially sure not to omit this very important set of tests. What good does it do to work hard on the *Quick Weight-Gain Program* if little animals inside your body are eating twice as fast as you are? If you have been to the Orient or the Middle East have your doctor include "flukes" in the diagnostic tests. (Maybe it's a good idea even if you haven't been to such strange places.)

I know what you're thinking. "How could a clean person like me get those awful things?" It's not your fault. This is getting to be a pretty messy world and parasites that used to live in the pestholes of faraway places are now sometimes right in your home town. So we have to find them and get rid of them so nothing stands in our way of putting on those precious pounds.

Of all the examinations, the test for diabetes is one of the most important. Since diabetes is basically a problem of metabolizing sugar and carbohydrates, if you have it you can eat like a horse and not put on an ounce. As a matter of fact, we doctors refer to the "triad of diabetes"—the three main symptoms—as "polydipsia, polyuria, and polyphagia." That's medical talk for: "drinking gallons of water, urinating gallons of water, and eating constantly." That's one of the common signs that a person suffers from the disease. Another source of unexplained weight loss is that old enemy, tuberculosis. But once your doctor puts you through these tests and gives you the go-ahead, you can start your weight-gain program with confidence.

One of the most effective tools in our program of weight gain is going to be a clear understanding of our personal metabolic rate. In the chemistry of our body, we "burn" our food just like a fireplace burns wood. And in the process of burning the food, like burning wood, oxygen is used up and carbon dioxide is produced. The amount of oxygen that we use to burn our food shows our "metabolic rate." The more oxygen we use, the higher our metabolic rate. There are a lot of things that determine that metabolic rate including exercise (increases it), emotions (can increase it or decrease it), and those things that affect women uniquely, like menstruation, pregnancy, and lactation.

Every person has their own unique individual rate of metabolism, which tells us two very important things: (1) How fast they convert their food into energy; (2) how fast they burn up that energy in their daily routine.

Once we get some idea of our metabolic rate, we can plan our weight-gain program around it and perhaps even do some very special things to adjust that rate to suit our needs. In general terms, body metabolism works like this:

Our organisms can be compared to an automobile engine. Every engine uses fuel at a different rate—some run fast and some run slow. Some bodies are like engines running at full throttle. They burn a lot of fuel (or food) and never have any excess energy left over to store as fat. These people are underweight and can never seem to gain weight. Other people have their body engines running at half speed. They don't burn up all the fuel (or food) they consume. They tend to gain weight because the excess food energy accumulates and is stored as fatty tissue.

There is one mysterious organ in the body that controls how fast our engine runs. That organ is the thyroid gland, a shield-shaped structure weighing about one ounce, located in the front of your neck, at about the level of the "Adam's apple." "Mysterious" is certainly the word for it. The thyroid takes iodine from the food you eat, combines it with an amino acid called "tyrosine," and converts it into two powerful hormones—thyroxine (or tetraiodothyronine) and triiodothyronine.[4] These two hormones are then carried to every remote corner of your body and precisely control the rate at which each cell and organ in your body operates. Like many other complex and mysterious aspects of our bodies nobody knows exactly how those hormones control our metabolic rate. But we do understand enough about it to accomplish our goal of gaining weight.

There is another very important gland at the base of our brain called the "pituitary gland." The pituitary does a lot of things but one important thing it does is produce a hormone called "thyroid-stimulating hormone," or "TSH" for short. TSH does exactly what its name says it does—it stimulates the thyroid to produce its hormones which are then poured into the blood and speed up our metabolism. The more thyroid hormone we have, the faster our motor runs and the harder it is to gain or maintain our weight. But there is a very special relationship between the thyroid and the pituitary. When the thyroid produces a lot of hormone, the pituitary senses it immediately and puts on the brakes.[5] But if the thyroid isn't secreting enough hormone, the pituitary sends it an urgent message ordering it to "get to work" and secrete more hormone. We can also take advantage of that mechanism to advance our weight-gaining campaign.

Let's take a few moments to see exactly what your metabolic rate is. Of course there are very precise—and expensive—medical tests that we can perform to get an exact measure of your metabolism. But for our needs, we can get a very good idea just by asking a few simple questions. Here they are:

1. Do your friends consider you to be a "nervous" person?
2. Do you tend to perspire even when other people in the room are comfortable?
3. Do you ever have palpitations (sudden rapid beating) of the heart?
4. Do you often feel restless and find it hard to sit still?

**5.** Do you find that sometimes your hands shake when you reach for something?

**6.** Do your eyes seem to be more prominent than other people's?

**7.** Do you have episodes of unexplained diarrhea?

If you answer "yes" to five or more of these questions, your thyroid may be significantly overactive. Before you go any further with your weight-gain program, see your doctor and have him carefully and precisely check the function of the gland. If your thyroid is seriously overactive, it needs to be corrected so that it won't interfere with the success of the *Quick Weight-Gain Program*. On the other hand if your thyroid is functioning relatively normally, you can expect maximum benefits from your weight-gain program. (If your thyroid is underactive you will probably be overweight and you won't be concerned about gaining still more weight.)

Most underweight people have relatively fast metabolic rates— within the normal range but still at the high end. That always makes it hard for them to gain and maintain weight. Wouldn't it be wonderful if we could make a simple adjustment to their thyroid gland and slow their metabolic rate just a little bit? If we could only find a way to safely slow down that master gland. Then their body "motors" would run a little more slowly and they could eat the same amount and gradually gain weight.

There are some very effective ways to slow down the thyroid gland and thus slow down the metabolic rate. Almost everyone that has it done, gains weight easily and effortlessly. One way is to operate on the neck and remove a big part of the gland. We're not going to do that! Another technique is to feed the patient iodine in a radioactive form that poisons the thyroid gland and slows its activity. You wouldn't be surprised if I told you we aren't going to do that either. We can also feed the patient large amounts of iodine that sort of "drowns" the thyroid in iodine and slows it down at the same time. That's not very appealing for a lot of reasons.

But what *can* we do? Well, there's another way to safely and effectively put the brakes on a mildly high-spirited thyroid. It's something that no one else has ever offered underweight people and it's going to be one of our important weapons in our "war on underweight." In chapter 5, we are going to safely and subtly coax our thyroid gland to calm down just enough to help us gain the weight we need. And that's going to make our whole project much easier and bring us to our ideal weight that much sooner. I know you'll be delighted with it!

## Chapter Two

# What They Never Told You About Underweight

**N**ow we're ready to clear the decks and get started! Let's begin by asking a question that will satisfy our curiosity and at the same time give us a very useful insight into some important secrets of gaining weight.

I'm sure you've noticed that almost everyone who stops smoking begins to put on weight immediately. But have you ever asked yourself "Why?" What is there about giving up those coffin nails that suddenly puts on the pounds? And more important, how can we use that knowledge to help us reach our goal of rapid and satisfying weight gain? Well, the standard explanations for weight gain among ex-smokers is that they crave sweets, or they need something to put into their mouth instead of cigarettes, or that they just feel nervous and eating calms them down. But those explanations don't seem to tell the whole story. If you think about it carefully there must be a deeper reason behind all of it. Of course there is and the real scientific explanation is a fascinating one. After years of very clever research, investigators have unraveled the whole story. Here it is:

Although many people don't realize it, our bodies use most of our energy just keeping all our organs working. Our heart has to pump gallons of blood, our lungs have to expand and contract, our digestive system has to work hard digesting our food—and everything else has to expand and contract, secrete and absorb, and constantly work at all the other 10,000 things that a busy body has to do.

About 75 percent of all the energy we use is devoted to just keeping everything working. We doctors call it the "Resting Energy Expenditure," or "REE."

If you smoke, you relentlessly zap your body with nicotine and all the rest of the 3,999 chemicals in cigarettes and significantly increase your REE. That means you have to eat just that much more to keep your weight where it is. It's like an automobile whose motor is racing even though the vehicle is parked motionless at the curb. It uses a lot of gasoline even though it doesn't go anywhere.

But as soon as you stop smoking, your REE drops dramatically. That is, the amount of energy you need just to keep your body working suddenly is *much less*. If you don't change anything else, you have to gain weight. How much? That depends on a lot of factors—we'll see about them as we go along. But in one big scientific study involving 6,580 men and women who stopped smoking, they gained an average of about 7 pounds *without even trying*. They just stopped smoking and the pounds came back on.[1]

In another carefully controlled study, people who stopped smoking were found to be eating 300 calories a day more *without being aware of it,* a mere 48 hours after they gave up cigarettes. Within a month they had put on about 3½ pounds.[2]

All in all, more than 80 percent of people who stopped smoking gained weight—some as much as 20 pounds. So, if you smoke, give yourself a big push in the right direction and throw those cigarettes away—forever! You'll be glad you did.

Now is also a good time to dispose of all those other bad habits that can interfere with our rapid and successful progress. The so-called recreational drugs—cocaine, heroin, amphetamines, ecstasy, "crack," and all the rest are the worst enemies of our weight-gain program. If you ever even thought of using them, stop right now! They will sabotage your chances to gain weight like nothing you've ever imagined. They will feed your entire body metabolism into a chemical meat-grinder and trash your chances of success once and for all.

Of the whole group, cocaine, "crack," and all amphetamine-related drugs are the worst offenders. They destroy your appetite and peel off the pounds like magic—*bad* magic. Remember, amphetamines are one of the drugs that overweight people use to reduce. So anyone who is really serious about gaining weight shouldn't even think about those drugs.

Strangely enough, alcohol is a different story. First of all, if you don't drink, there's no reason to start just to help yourself gain weight. But if you do drink moderately, there are some interesting ways that you can choose what and when you drink to help put on weight. Alcoholic beverages, judiciously used, can assist you in your program. *But don't start drinking just for that.* And remember, drinking too much can backfire and interfere with successful weight gain. The full explanation, with instructions, is in chapters 4 and 9.

As we get our weight-gain program underway, it will be very useful if we take a moment to review what happens to our food when we eat it. It will help us understand what's really going on inside of us as well as aid us in planning successful strategy. At the same time, we'll make an amazing discovery or two.

The three basic components of the food we eat—and the elements that are essential for the health and maintenance of our bodies—are protein, carbohydrate, and fat.

An example of protein is meat, fish, or chicken. Carbohydrate consists of two kinds of foods—starches like bread, potatoes, and pasta plus sugars like honey, cane sugar, etc. Fat is cooking oil like corn oil and the solid fat on meat. Actually we *almost* never find these three elements in pure form. Meat has protein and fat—but no carbohydrate. Eggs have all three components. A baked potato also has all three elements—fat, protein, and carbohydrate, but, of course, in different proportions. Table sugar is pure carbohydrate. As we go along we'll take a look at various foods to see whether their combinations of these three vital elements fit in with our weight-gain plans.

As we go through our day we select the foods we consume in a sort of random way. A lot of what we eat—and when we eat it—is determined by habit, by chance, and by what we've read in magazines or seen on television. Look at the typical American breakfast:

1 glass of orange juice—or powdered orange drink
1 slice of toasted bread with butter or margarine
1 small bowl of breakfast cereal (composed of mixed
    processed grains, often with sugar already added)
1 cup of coffee with sugar and milk or cream or cream
    substitute

Sometimes that meal includes an egg—for those who don't worry about the *supposed* effect on their blood cholesterol.

That same meal is consumed by tens of millions of people day in and day out. As many as 17 percent of those people are underweight and most of those want to gain weight. Unfortunately, eating *that* kind of breakfast isn't going to help them very much. In spite of that, that's been their breakfast ever since childhood and that's what they eat!

The same is true of the typical lunch. It usually works out to something like this:

1 sandwich (sometimes 2, consisting of 2 slices of bread
    with meat, chicken, or fish, sometimes combined
    with processed cheese. It may also contain lettuce,
    mayonnaise, butter, etc.)
1 cup of coffee or a carbonated soft drink
Dessert, consisting of a piece of pie, a piece of cake, or
    a dish of ice cream

Other variations might include a hamburger on a bun (sometimes with processed cheese) or some pizza.

Most lunches are eaten at work or school and are based as much on convenience as nutrition. Your chances of gaining weight on the usual American lunch are about the same as being run over by a cable car in San Francisco on Christmas Day while carrying an Easter bunny under each arm during a monsoon.

Supper is even a worse bet. The standard American evening

meal is meat, potatoes, and two vegetables, plus dessert. Sometimes soup finds its way on to the menu and occasionally pizza or hamburgers. But the meal is usually tedious and unappealing—and useless for weight gain.

After dinner there is television and snacks. The snacks are basically fried starch concoctions—potato chips, corn chips, and variations on that theme. By their design they are almost useless for gaining weight. Here's the great paradox of the American diet—and at the same time, the challenge that we are going to overcome. The traditional American diet is ideal for gaining weight—*if you want to stay thin!* And it is almost worthless for gaining weight if you are underweight! One reason is that the typical diet has far too much protein—and we'll discover in detail how protein sabotages weight gain before this chapter is over. In addition, overweight people manipulate their carbohydrate stores in a way that underweight people have never thought of. If those who are underweight learn to manage their carbohydrate metabolism the way their heavier brothers and sisters do, they will put on weight that much more easily. But we're going to take care of that too in the pages that follow.

But right now we're going to briefly review how our food is digested. It will help us to understand what's really happening inside us when we eat—and it will help us make the best choices for putting the weight on. It may be different from what you learned back in school because there have been a lot of new discoveries since then. Here it is—the short version:

Although we don't usually think about it that way, digestion begins as soon as we start to chew our first bite of food. A digestive enzyme in our saliva called ''ptyalin'' starts to work digesting the carbohydrate in what we eat. Then we swallow the food, now reduced to a moist mass, and it slides down to our stomach. Then a powerful acid, hydrochloric acid, acts on it along with another enzyme called ''pepsin.'' By that time whatever we have eaten is pretty much in a liquid form. As it is moved out of the stomach by muscular action, the liquid enters the duodenum, which is the beginning of the small intestine.

At that point enzymes from the pancreas are squirted into the food. These enzymes digest the protein and carbohydrate in whatever we have eaten. At the same time, bile from the gall bladder is added to digest the fat.

That's where most of the digestive part takes place. The food is broken down into basic components—fat, protein, and carbohydrate—so it can be used by the body. For the remainder of its trip through the digestive system, absorption is the key word. In the rest of the small intestine—about 16½ feet of it—fat, protein, and carbohydrate are absorbed selectively.

But once these basic components are absorbed, it really gets interesting. That's the part of digestion that we call "utilization." The various components of our food are used by our body for energy—to operate our organs and to just move around. That's interesting. But whatever we eat that is not used for energy is stored—and stored eventually as that extra weight we want so badly. And for those of us who want to gain weight, the storage process is where the action is!

The way our bodies deal with fat, protein, and carbohydrate is fascinating—and almost totally overlooked in the usual books. It is tremendously important for us to be aware of it since the secrets of the way our food is utilized hold the secrets to fast and easy weight gain.

Although few people realize it, the protein you eat—eggs, cheese, porterhouse steak—can be quickly and easily transformed by your body into fat or carbohydrate. And the carbohydrate you eat can be just as quickly and easily transformed into fat. Even more interesting, the fat can be converted to carbohydrate. The only thing that can't happen—ever—is for either fat or carbohydrate to be converted to protein. So to summarize, protein can be converted to anything and fat and carbohydrate can be exchanged for each other, but nothing can be made into protein. The only way you can get it is to eat it.

What does it all mean to us? Well, it means a lot. For all practical purposes, the only way we can store long-term energy is in the form of fat. Plants, on the other hand, can store energy as carbohydrate. That's what a potato is, for example. It is the root of a plant that stores its energy as carbohydrate. Plants can do that because they don't have to walk around. Stored carbohydrate molecules are surrounded by water and they are very heavy—if humans stored energy as carbohydrates, the average person would weigh 950 pounds and be shaped like a potato.

By contrast, storing energy as fat is wonderfully efficient. You can pack a tremendous amount of energy into a very small space and then use the energy when you need it. For example, 1 gram of carbohydrate burned (metabolized) in your body produces about 4 calories of energy. But when 1 gram of fat is metabolized, it produces about 9 calories, or more than twice as much (1 gram of protein metabolized in your body produces about 4 calories—the same as carbohydrate).

Since we want to put on weight, we really want to put on fat—with whatever additional muscle tissue we can manage. We want to round out our bodies, add the bulk that we are missing, and look and feel healthy. If we have a low Body Mass Index (BMI), that's an indication of a deficiency of body fat. So we want to convert as much protein and carbohydrate to fat. At the same time— and we'll see very soon how vital this is—we want to prevent at all costs the conversion of fat to carbohydrate.

Why? Because when fat is converted to carbohydrate, it is poured into the blood as sugar and immediately burned up. Remember, our bodies can utilize carbohydrate as fuel. So if we are going to gain weight we have a double mission: to add to our fat stores and to protect them against the danger of being converted to carbohydrate and instantly burned away.

Here is the key to the whole process—and one of the important keys to weight gain. During digestion, carbohydrate is converted to sugar and deposited in the liver as a substance called "glycogen." Glycogen is really a series of simple sugars hooked together to form a very special and temporary kind of carbohydrate. It's a carbohydrate that can be very quickly utilized without having to go through the tedious process of being digested again. Glycogen is easily converted into simple sugars and can be poured into the blood on short notice to be burned up for fast energy.

But if we can load up the liver with so much glycogen that it can't possibly hold any more, the rest of the carbohydrate we consume has no place to go and *must be converted to fat*. That's going to be one of our basic strategies: to pack so much glycogen into the liver that the next spoonful of carbohydrate we eat—and all the spoonfuls and forkfuls after that—are *immediately and directly* deposited as fat.

We want this process of fat formation to go as quickly and as smoothly as possible. We don't want anything to interfere with it. And there are two traps that can divert the carbohydrate from its destination—the liver. Both of them are most threatening at one specific time—right after eating. The traps are "exercise" and what we doctors call "Specific Dynamic Action," or "SDA" for short.

Here's the way it works:

After you eat, as your food is being digested, the carbohydrate is converted to sugar and deposited in your liver as glycogen. To gain weight we're trying to fill that liver right to the brim with all the glycogen we can. As soon as the liver is full, all the rest of what we eat should go directly to fat—that extra weight we're so eager to put on. But as soon as we start to exercise our body gets a signal to pull the glycogen out of the liver and pour it into the bloodstream as sugar—to provide the energy we need to move our muscles. Once we start to move around, we pull that precious glycogen out of the liver and what we eat from then on has to go back into the liver to replenish it. The worst part is that we have hardly any reserve of glycogen. Even if we fill our liver up to the brim, it will only contain about 4 percent glycogen—barely a 24-hour supply. So if we move around a lot after meals, we dump the glycogen out of our liver, and whatever we eat after that can't go to adding weight. It has to go to refilling the empty liver.

That means that our first rule of weight gain—even before we start talking about exactly which foods to eat and how to eat them—is this:

(1) Do not engage in any exercise for at least 2 hours after eating. It would be even better to avoid any movement for 2 hours but that's obviously not practical for everyone. If you're at home, it's a good idea to lie down immediately after each meal for at least 30 minutes. Watch TV, read, listen to music, take a nap—whatever you enjoy the most. Let your liver fill with glycogen so that the rest of your food will be diverted to weight gain.

If you're at work in an office, try and sit as calmly as possible, without any exertion or unnecessary movement. If your job keeps you in motion, do the best you can to minimize your exertion but be sure and rest after each meal when you're not working.

If this technique seems simple, it's because it is simple. The problem is that no one has taken the time and the interest to analyze the problem of underweight. For the past 50 years the vast resources of the medical profession have been devoted basically to taking weight off. No one—until now—has cared about the 48 million underweight Americans. The reason is totally understandable—and totally misguided.

So much of our medical resources have been devoted to taking off weight because of the mistaken belief that overweight people get sick more often and at a higher rate than those who are underweight. The truth is that in 9 out of 10 scientific studies, *underweight people run a greater risk of death[3] than those who are overweight.*[4] According to a medical study of the World Health Organization underweight men have 20 times more chance of dying than overweight men. The Canadian Ministry of Health, in their research, found underweight men die at twice the rate of overweight men.[5]

After more than 5 years of careful study and after reviewing more than 1200 scientific papers on all aspects of human digestion and metabolism, I can safely say that I have uncovered, catalogued, and perfected the scientific secrets of gaining weight. Something apparently as simple as lying down after each meal has a solid scientific basis and works wonders. But that's only the beginning. The second rule of weight gain is equally fascinating.

(2) Always wear a sweater or jacket while eating. Never eat a

meal in a cold place or where you will be chilled. Ideally, you should take a hot shower or spend at least 15 minutes in warm surroundings immediately after eating.

Does that sound unusual too? Sure it does—because no one, until now, has taken the time and effort to scientifically analyze the most important and yet little-known factors that control and affect our body weight. Here's the explanation:

When we eat, our food is burned in our bodies, just like coal or wood, to produce energy. That energy can be used to move our muscles—or it can be used to heat our bodies and keep us warm. The energy that is not used—the energy that we don't have to spend—is stored as fat. And that's what we're after!

Everyone has heard the word ''calorie'' in relation to weight—especially those who are trying to lose weight. In scientific terms the heat from 80 calories will melt 1 gram (or about 1/30 of an ounce) of ice; boiling the same amount of water requires 540 calories. Calories are very interesting in another way since a ''calorie'' is not a calorie.[6] What we so calmly refer to as a ''calorie'' is really one thousand of them. Since human beings produce such vast amounts of heat, we need to express their energy usage in units that are 1000 times as large as regular calories. We call these units ''large calories.'' So when you see a piece of cake listed in one of those diet books at 800 calories, it really contains 800,000 calories! Those little details are more curiosities of scientific history. But what follows is a cold, hard fact that we can immediately use to put on more pounds.

In order for a person to maintain his weight exactly where it happens to be, he must consume on the average about 1.5 calories (of the large kind) each and every minute—day and night. In a practical sense that means two things for us:

We must consume enough calories when we do eat to make up for the time when we are not eating. That requires a certain amount of dedication plus taking advantage of the broad collection of hints, helpful techniques, diet suggestions, and menu plans in the chapters that follow.

And vitally important, we must make sure that we lose as little heat as possible so that as much as possible of the food energy goes to weight instead of being dissipated into thin air.

That's where "Specific Dynamic Action" comes in. Specific Dynamic Action is a strange and mysterious event that happens to everyone every day of their life. It consists of a tremendously dramatic metabolic explosion that happens several times a day—but no one in the world has ever been able to explain it!

In spite of decades of investigation no one can tell us why our metabolism suddenly and uncontrollably erupts like a renegade volcano. Although it is critically important in every weight-gain program, you have never seen it mentioned before in any weight-management book ever published! Here is the full story now, for the first time:

The next time you are feeling a bit chilly when it's time to sit down to a meal, don't put on a sweater. Just pull your chair up to the table and eat. Within a few moments you will actually begin to feel warmer, and if it is a heavy meal, you may actually have to open a window. The simple act of eating produces a sudden burst of heat of metabolic activity that can actually make you perspire. The rate at which your body is utilizing the food which you have just eaten suddenly explodes! From one moment to the next, the rate at which you burn up your food increases as much as 30 percent—just like that! To make things worse, the effect can last 8 hours or so after you eat. The Specific Dynamic Action supercharges your metabolic rate all day—and sometimes all night. The scientific explanation? No one knows!

But I do know this: it is a deadly trap for anyone who wants to gain weight. Look at what happens. Say an average person produces about 75 calories an hour in heat—just to keep his body working. Those calories have to come from somewhere and they come from two places. They come from the food you eat and from your own body stores of energy; that is, from your body weight in the form of fat. If you produce more energy in heat than you eat in food, you use up your body fat fast. That's a problem that everyone who is underweight faces every day. But suddenly we have to take into account that monster of Specific Dynamic Action. No one has ever told you about it—much less how to protect yourself against it—but it eats up your calories and uses up your precious body weight every day of your life.

Here's a typical example. Let's say that you consume 100 grams of protein at a meal to gain the benefit of about 410 calories—an important amount if you are trying to gain weight. You're burning up 75 calories an hour just to keep your body working and those 410 calories will hold you for about 5½ hours—with luck. But suddenly your luck runs out. Without any warning—and against your will—your metabolic rate suddenly jumps up to 97.5 calories an hour! Now that same amount of food will only keep you going 4 hours and 12 minutes. After that, you start gobbling up your own body weight just to keep functioning. No one knows why, but for some reason protein speeds your rate of metabolism and drains your reserves of body weight. It's like being down to your last few drops of gasoline and racing your car as fast as you can to the gas station before you run out of gas. You eat protein to gain weight and the protein makes your body shed that weight faster than you are putting it on!

What's the solution? Well, the first step is to know that it's happening. Otherwise you can eat and eat and eat and wonder why you never seem to put on weight. And that's why you hear so many underweight people say, "I can't understand it! I eat all the time and yet I never can manage to gain an ounce!"

The next step is to learn more about the problem. Protein is the worst culprit—it raises our metabolic rate 30 percent. But if we eat carbohydrate, we only increase the rate at which we burn our food by 6 percent. And if we emphasize fat, we only burn away an extra 4 percent of what we eat. So our defense against the destructive force of Specific Dynamic Action is really twofold:

1. Prevent the heat loss after every meal because heat is energy and energy lost is weight lost.
2. Design our diet to avoid as much as possible that

energy-wasting protein. We'll cover that in detail when we come to the exciting menus and diet plans in chapters 14 and 15.

But in the meantime, here are a couple of important and useful hints. The average person in the United States eats about 3½ ounces of fat a day—that's about 30 percent of his or her calories. He or she also consumes about 20 ounces of carbohydrate daily, made up of about 60 percent starch and about 40 percent various forms of sugar. That's about 60 percent of the daily caloric intake. That diet also includes about 2½ ounces of protein per day or about 10 percent of the diet calories. (These are approximate values since individual variations are substantial.)

With what we already know, any diet that has that kind of distribution of calories between fat, protein, and carbohydrate should start all the warning bells ringing. That 10 percent protein is generating tremendous amounts of Specific Dynamic Action heat and costing us vast numbers of calories that we could otherwise dedicate to putting on weight. In a real sense, our potential weight gain is going up the chimney in useless heat. Let's take another look at our previous example just to see how bad it really is:

If a person gives off 75 calories per hour in heat and the protein which he consumes raises his heat production 30 percent, he suddenly starts to burn off 97.25 calories an hour. In a 24-hour period that's 2,334 calories that he is losing. One pound of extra weight (as fat) requires 3,500 extra calories above your daily energy requirements. That 534 calories per day you lose from the protein-triggered Specific Dynamic Action (SDA for short) robs you of about 2½ ounces of potential weight gain every 24 hours. That's a little over a pound a week that Specific Dynamic Action can steal from you.

Now, most people aren't losing a pound a week from SDA-produced heat loss. But that just may be the pound that they can't gain. It's like trying to cool your house on a scorching summer afternoon with the air conditioner on full and the windows wide open.

So, what do we do? Well, we can't stop the SDA from happening. Since no one knows why it happens, certainly they don't know how to turn it off. But we can carefully conserve our body heat just after eating—at the moment when SDA does its greatest damage. That sudden burst of heat that everyone feels halfway or so into a meal is like a leak in our gasoline tank.

We'll also see how to select foods that minimize the damage done by SDA. Remember that carbohydrate only raises our metabolism by 6 percent and fat only cranks up our metabolic rate by a mere 4 percent. That means under the same circumstances, using the previous example, if we eat fat, SDA only steals 80 calories a day—that adds up to cheating us out of about 2 ounces a week. That's not good but it's better than a whole pound.

If it's carbohydrate that sets off our SDA, it only burns up about 120 calories a day and steals 3 ounces a week that would otherwise go to building up our weight. We can deal with that much more easily than having a whole pound slip away from us every 7 days.

So now we have two brand-new arrows in our quiver—we know that we have the power to alter our body's metabolic rate at least two ways. First, we can redirect the flow of carbohydrate from stored glycogen into stored fat. And second, we can stem the loss of weight by keeping our calories from being drained away into the air as heat.

As we turn the page to the never-before-published (except in obscure medical texts) details in chapter 3, we'll see some very excellent and very specific techniques that will help us translate our new knowledge into new pounds. Here we go!

## Chapter Three

# How to Gain with "Friendly Fat"

**A**ndrea shifted uncomfortably in her chair.

"What's the trouble, Andrea?"

She smiled. "You know what the trouble is, Doctor! You have a nice office but there just isn't enough padding in the chairs for us skinny folks and we don't have any padding of our own! But it's another problem that I'm concerned with."

"What's that?"

"Well, you know that I'm here to gain weight but I certainly don't want to be fat!"

She said the word "fat" as if it were another word for "flesh-eating bacteria."

"What do you mean?"

"It's simple. I manage a chain of coffee bars and I'm always in contact with the public. Now I hate to be thin—and I know you're going to solve that problem for me. But I certainly don't want to be bursting out of my clothes and overflowing with blubber!"

It was my turn to smile.

"I don't think there's any danger of that, Andrea. Let me explain it this way."

I picked up her medical chart. "I see here you're 25 years old, you weigh 109 pounds, and you're 5 feet 7 inches tall. That means you have a body mass index of 17.14. The minimum BMI for your height and weight and age is about 19. Let's call it 19.5 to give you a little extra reserve. That means you should weigh about 124 pounds. If you're 15 pounds underweight, it's no wonder you were shifting around in your chair—you don't have enough fat on your bottom to cushion you when you sit down.''

Andrea laughed. ''Okay, Doctor, you can put a little more fat down there to cushion me when I sit. But I don't want a fat belly or a double chin. Can't you just help me to gain weight but not put on fat?''

''Andrea, just about the only way you can put on weight without adding fat is to swallow fish sinkers. There is one exception, and we'll tell you how to do that in chapter 5—but for all practical purposes, your weight gain is going to be fat—and that's not really bad news. This is how it works:

''Your body is composed of many different organs—heart, lungs, kidneys, and all the rest. Obviously we can't increase the weight of those structures, nor would we want to if we could. Then there's skin and bones and connective tissue. We can't really make those heavier, either. What's left? Well, there's muscle. We can add a little bit of weight in the form of muscular development—and we're going to do that in chapter 5—to round out your figure and even make you a little sexier, if that's what you want.''

Andrea's face lighted up. ''I'd like to meet the girl who doesn't want to be at least a little sexier!''

''Fine. But that still leaves us with a problem. If we can't add bone or skin or organs, how do we gain weight? That's right— adding fat is the only way. But it isn't a bad idea.''

''But say we put on those 15 pounds. What can I expect to see?''

''Well, it all depends on whether you're a man or a woman. Since you're a woman you can expect to deposit some of the fat on your hips and buttocks.''

''Thank goodness! My skirts will finally fit!''

''And you'll be able to sit in my office chairs without suffering. At the same time, your breasts will fill out—after all, they are basically fat. And your body contours will become rounder instead of angular, the way they are now. You'll have some fat deposited on the calves of your legs and your thighs."

"But I won't get chubby?"

I had to smile again. "Not with a BMI of 19.5 and a total body weight of 124 pounds! Besides, the Quick Weight-Gain Program is designed with built-in protective mechanisms specifically to prevent anything like that from happening. Don't worry."

Just as we are going to gain weight by depositing fat, we are going to gain weight by increasing the amount of fat we consume in our daily diet. And the first step is to get rid of a big bugaboo: Fear-of-Fat. For more than 25 years we have been bombarded by articles, books, and television commercials warning us about the dangers of F-A-T.[1] The net result is that today everyone is pressured more and more to eliminate every last trace of fat from their diet. That's excellent advice if you're 5 feet tall and you weigh 200 pounds. It's also good advice if you eat three fat pork chops every night for dinner and your cholesterol is over 350. But fat in and of itself won't do you a bit of harm. But don't believe it just because I say it. Listen to what the Food and Nutrition Board of the National Research Council of the U.S. National Academy of Sciences said. They concluded that the evidence warrants *no specific recommendations about limiting dietary fat intake for healthy people.*[2]

Let's take a moment to review the basic facts about fat. In recent years tens of thousands of pages have been written about fat—saturated fat, unsaturated fat, polyunsaturated fat, hydrogenated fat, partially hydrogenated fat, and all the rest. Here's the real story about fat—as it affects us on the Quick Weight-Gain Program.

What we call fat is found in our diets as both "fats" and "oils." Nutritionally they are the same except that "fats" are solid at room temperature and "oils" are liquid at room temperature. For example, corn oil is an "oil" and chicken fat is a "fat" but nutritionally they are basically the same—with one difference that we will see in a moment. (For simplicity we will call both fats and oils "fat" from now on.) The immense controversy about "saturated" versus "unsaturated'' fats is based on the way that the atoms that make up fats are hooked together. Fats are all constructed around one basic design—a central atom of carbon hooked into several atoms of hydrogen. It looks something like this:

Hydrogen

|

Hydrogen - Carbon - Hydrogen

|

Hydrogen

If the carbon atoms have soaked up all the hydrogen they can, the fat is called ''saturated.'' If the carbon atoms still have room to grab more hydrogen atoms, the fat is ''unsaturated.'' That's it! Animal fat—like chicken fat, pig fat (lard), and beef fat (tallow)—is ''saturated'' and considered ''bad'' because it is thought to increase ''bad'' cholesterol deposits in your arteries. (To make matters more complicated, there is also ''good'' cholesterol that is considered okay. Fortunately we don't have to get involved in all the ins and outs of that controversy here. We just want to put on some weight!)

On the other hand, corn oil, olive oil, safflower oil, soybean oil, and most of the liquid-at-room-temperature fats have a lot of ''unsaturated'' components. The exception is what we call ''tropical oils''—including palm kernel oil, palm oil, and coconut oil. They have a lot of saturated components and are thought to be about as unattractive cholesterol-wise as animal fats.

And just to prove that the fat controversy is not as simple as it looks, take the example of margarine. To produce margarine, food processors bubble hydrogen gas through ''unsaturated'' soybean oil (which is supposed to be ''good'' in relation to forming cholesterol) to make it solid at room temperature so it looks and tastes more or less like butter. So you have perfection: a ''good'' unsaturated fat that looks and tastes like butter—a delicious ''bad'' saturated fat. One little problem: all that hydrogen converts the liquid ''unsaturated'' soybean oil into a fairly saturated solid fat. So you end up with a product that isn't that much better—in terms of saturation—than plain old butter.

Why go all through this? Because anyone who really wants to gain weight is going to have to include a fair amount of fat in their diet. Fat is concentrated energy in storage. If you want to gain weight, you have to take the stored fat from somewhere else—a plant or an animal—and transfer it to your own storage depots. Since fat has gotten a lot of confusing publicity *we want to feel confident that nothing in this diet is going to do us any harm.* So it's worth taking a few moments to get a clear idea of what fat is really composed of and where the hazards—*if there are any hazards*—lie. As the opinion of the Food and Nutrition Board of the National Research Council of the U.S. National Academy of Sciences that we just mentioned emphasizes, there is no convincing proof that consuming fat of *any kind* will really do you harm.

However, in this diet, to be absolutely supersafe, we divide our fat consumption sensibly between animal fats and vegetable fats. While it is almost certainly harmless for someone who is underweight to eat any kind of fat, on the Quick Weight-Gain Program we will be absolutely supercautious and still gain all the weight we want.

And prepare yourself for the inevitable. One evening you will be eating dinner and some well-meaning friend will look at your plate, make a face, and ask, "Oh, why are you eating *all that fat?*"

Just smile and reply, "I'm eating carefully calculated amounts of high-energy fat because I'd like to keep on living. Did you know that the World Health Organization has proved that being underweight increases your risk of death by 2,000 percent?"[3]

And it's true. If all the stories about fat consumption causing heart attacks are true, you can expect to have trouble after about 48 years on a high-fat diet. (Heart attacks begin to show up in significant numbers after the age of fifty or so.) Since you should gain an average of a pound a week on the Quick Weight-Gain Program, even if you put on as much as 30 pounds you'll be on a fat-enhanced diet for barely over 6 months. That leaves you 47½ years to go before you can start worrying about the bad effects of fat.[4]

Now let's ask the first of two very important questions: "Why are adequate fat stores so important to our health?"

There are three answers. First, adding fat to our bodies is much more than just improving our appearance. Fat is the reserve of energy that powers our body. If we are injured in a serious accident or if we suffer a severe illness, we have to survive completely or partially on our fat stores until our body can resume its normal functions. Secondly, fat plays a key role in the metabolism of our most important vitamins. Vitamins A, D, E, and K are vital for the functioning of our bodies. They are all fat soluble and require fat stores for their storage and utilization. Thirdly and more subtle—but just as important—is the role of fat deposits in the metabolism of basic hormones. Just one example: women with adequate fat stores have fewer problems in the menopause because their extra fat helps preserve their supply of estrogen, the main female sex hormone.[5]

The second question is, "Why is it so important for us to eat foods containing fat if we want to gain weight?"

The answer to that question lies in three magic numbers: 4-4-9. Remember back in chapter 1 when we saw that 1 gram of carbohydrate supplies 4 calories, and 1 gram of protein also supplies 4 grams of calories? That was when we saw that *1 gram of fat gives us 9 calories of energy.* (The precise figures are 4.1 for carbohydrate, 4.1 for protein, and a whopping 9.3 for fat.)

That means that if we just eat the same amount of food—substituting fat for other components as much as reasonably possible—we will more than double our caloric intake and put on weight that much faster. We can gain twice as much weight in the same time or reach our goal twice as fast. In addition, we can avoid a lot of problems, including putting our kidneys at risk with an excessive consumption of protein.

Let's take a look at the caloric advantages of adding fat to our diet. The figures are really impressive:

For example, one serving of spaghetti with tomato sauce and cheese will give you 104 calories. (Let's call a "serving" 3½ ounces—and from now on we'll use that amount as our standard serving for comparison purposes. When you sit down to the table, of course, you can eat as much as you want.) To put on that 1 pound of weight, you will have to eat 7⅓ pounds of spaghetti. But try pizza with cheese topping—another Italian delight—and you'll get 236 calories in the same-size serving. That means you'll only have to eat 3¼ pounds of pizza to put on that pound. Of course you wouldn't have to eat all that pizza at one sitting. All you would have to do is consume that amount of pizza above and beyond the basic number of calories you need to maintain your weight. For example, if you eat 2,000 calories a day and you don't gain and you don't lose, then 3½ ounces of pizza a day—extra—would put on an additional pound in two weeks, all other things being equal. Of course these are just illustrations. We'll get down to the detailed menus and recipes in chapters 14 and 15.

There's another problem that we have to deal with in our campaign to put on weight—but don't worry—we have the solution for that one too. It's one of the problems with fat that we are going to show you how to overcome in chapter 6. Fat has what we doctors call a high "satiety" value. "Satiety" comes from the Latin word *satis,* which means "enough." And that's it. More than any other category of food, fat has the ability—when it reaches a certain concentration in your bloodstream—to make you want to *stop eating.*

No one knows exactly how it works but there seems to be a detector somewhere in the brain that measures the amount of fat that we are consuming. When we get to a certain amount—different for different people—the brain screams: "Yuck! No more fat!" And then we don't want any more fat. If we ignore the alarm and keep trying to eat more fat, our stomach seconds the brain's complaint and that's the moment when even the most determined eater gets the idea. That's why the ultimate example is such a difficult one to achieve. It's this: If you could consume 3½ ounces of pure fat in the form of pure oil, you would get 884 calories. That means a pound of oil would put on about a pound of weight. But you can't do it just like that. Your brain and your stomach won't let you. (Although there is a trick that will help overcome "satiety" problems. We'll talk about that farther on.)

So one of our goals is going to be getting fat and other high-calorie items into our diet without ever tripping the "satiety" alarm. Actually it's not going to be very hard. Even better, it's going to be interesting, exciting, and enjoyable.

One thing that will help us a lot is to become "fat detectives." So many of our overweight friends have developed the detection of fat into a fine art. All they have to do is bite into any item on their plate. If it contains even a micro-ounce of fat, they make a face and shout, "Ugh! Fat!" We'd like to be able to do the same thing, only when we detect a generous content of fat our faces should light up as we announce, "Ahhh! Fat!" These days we live in a period of "food hysteria." It's a "low-fat," "low-calorie," "lite" world. But that's exactly what we're struggling against. In a real sense, we have to watch how everyone else eats and basically do the opposite. We want to create a "high-fat," a "high-calorie," a "heavy" environment. So think "fat." As a good start, here's a preliminary list of a few common high-fat foods—including some that we may not have actually thought of as "high fat."

To help us along, we're going to grade each category of fat-containing food as to its real value to us. There are going to be some surprises, as we will see. Here's the code:

☺ Good source of calories because of its fat content
☺ Even better source of calories because of its fat content
☹ Not as good as it seems for special reasons.

☺ Nuts: (except Macadamia) [peanuts, almonds, cashews, mixed nuts, etc.] 1 ounce of nuts adds about 170–180 calories but there's an interesting twist. The "dry roasted" nuts—presumably cooked without oil—only save a skimpy 10 calories or so. But nuts also have something very special going for them, something that will help you in an amazing way to gain that weight—and something that no one has ever told you about before. The full story is in chapter 5 and when you see it you'll be amazed and delighted!

☺ Macadamia Nuts: That's where we hit the jackpot. Macadamias weigh in at 207 calories per ounce. And hickory nuts—if you can find them—are a good 200 calories per ounce. Not bad.

☹ Potato chips: Potato chips are a two-edged sword for us. While they have a respectable caloric count—160 calories or so per ounce—they also fill you up very fast, which keeps you from eating too many. One reason is that they have a lot of starch and also tons of salt. The starch fills you up too fast. The salt makes you thirsty, you drink a lot of liquid, and you feel full. That's what we want to avoid on the Quick Weight-Gain Program—a feeling of fullness. We want to be able to put all those wonderful calories to work for us without ever feeling stuffed or bloated or overly full. The same problem arises with corn chips, and all the rest of the fried starchy snacks.

☺ However—as always—there is a way out. If we combine the chips with dips, then we can up the calories and avoid the problems.

To get the benefit of high-calorie dips you can start with this quick and easy approach. Take a cup of sour cream—470 calories—and add a package of "dip mix." You know the kind I mean—it comes in blue cheese and onion flavors and a dozen more varieties. Just make sure you get a high-calorie brand—say about 130 calories per ounce. Add it to the sour cream, and you have at least 600 calories right there. Eat it slowly as a snack with an ounce of corn chips or potato chips at 160 calories and you have 760 nice calories to help you on your way. If you just have a snack like that about 5 times (eating right the rest of the time too) you can put on 1 extra pound.

☺ Hot dogs (frankfurters, wieners): Since there is a lot of variation in the ingredients, the caloric value of these sausages varies wildly. But if you read labels carefully, you can find single sausages that have as much as 280 calories or so. Add 2 tablespoons of mustard at

30 calories, 4 pieces of sweet pickle at 50 calories, ½ ounce of melted cheese (if you like) at 50 calories, and a bun at 120 calories and you have a nice 530-calorie package.

☺ Cheese Snacks: Cheese is a funny food. Some cheeses have a lot of calories and some are calorie poor. Your best bet is among the "cheese foods"—check the label carefully for the product with the highest calorie count. These are the combinations of soft cheese with things like pimento and bacon and salami. They run about 100 calories per ounce and are easy to eat. For maximum benefit put as much cheese as you can on the smallest possible cracker. That gives you the most fat for each bite.

That's just a tiny selection of the high-fat foods that are going to be very useful to us as we go along. Now let's look at one of the important secrets of weight gain.

What we are going to do is turn the tables on the weight-reduction crowd. They specialize in meals that look the same as normal meals but have many of the calories drained out of them. For example, at lunch they might eat the following:

A glass of fat-free milk, a sandwich with "diet" bread, very low fat turkey slices, lo-cal mayonnaise, no-fat salad dressing, and a fat-free dessert.

Their secret is they get just about as full and just about as satisfied as if they had eaten a normal meal. But the calorie count for that lunch is a mere 336 calories.

## THE I-WANT-TO-LOSE-WEIGHT LUNCH

| | | |
|---|---|---|
| 2 slices of diet bread | @ 35 calories | 70 calories |
| 8 ounces of nonfat milk | @ 80 calories | 80 calories |
| I ounce sliced turkey | @ 45 calories | 45 calories |
| 3 tablespoons lo-cal mayonnaise | @ 10 calories | 30 calories |
| 3 tablespoons no-fat salad dressing | @ 10 calories | 30 calories |
| 3 leaves lettuce | @ 2 calories | 6 calories |
| I strawberry gelatin dessert | @ 75 calories | 75 calories |

Now let's look at a normal lunch.

## THE I-JUST-WANT-LUNCH LUNCH

| | | |
|---|---|---|
| 2 slices of regular bread | @ 60 calories | 120 calories |
| 8 ounces full-fat milk | @ 160 calories | 160 calories |
| 1 ounce ham | @ 70 calories | 70 calories |
| 3 tablespoons mayonnaise | @ 100 calories | 300 calories |
| 3 tablespoons no-fat salad dressing | @ 80 calories | 240 calories |
| 3 leaves lettuce | @ 2 calories | 6 calories |
| 1 slice of chocolate cake | @ 175 calories | 175 calories |

That's a total of 1,071 calories at lunchtime. And remember, the chap who ate the "low-calorie" lunch should feel as full (well, almost as full) as the one who ate the normal lunch. Both of them had their *one chance* to eat lunch that day and that's the amount of calories they absorbed.

But we can do better! If we only eat the same bulk of food—so that we don't feel stuffed or overfilled—we can squeeze in more calories per ounce of lunch. Remember, we only have one chance to gain weight at lunch that day! With no extra effort, here's what we can do:

## THE QUICK WEIGHT-GAIN PROGRAM LUNCH

| | | |
|---|---|---|
| 2 slices of white bread | @ 80 calories | 160 calories |
| 1 8-ounce milk shake (from mix) | @ 290 calories | 290 calories |
| 1 ounce hard salami | @ 120 calories | 120 calories |
| 3 tablespoons mayonnaise | @ 100 calories | 300 calories |
| 3 tablespoons salad dressing | @ 100 calories | 300 calories |
| 3 leaves lettuce | @ 2 calories | 6 calories |
| 1 apple turnover with ½ cup ice cream | @ 420 calories | 420 calories |

We're now up to 1,596 calories—an increase of 526 calories with hardly any extra effort. That's a 49 percent increase over the "average" lunch, and if we only manage a similar advantage every day—just at lunch—we should gain a pound in just under a week. As you can see, if we approach putting on weight systematically, it isn't going to be that difficult.

And if we analyze the caloric gains we have made in the Quick Weight-Gain Program, we'll see that a lot of them are simply from increasing the amount of fat in an ordinary meal. (We've also increased the amount of carbohydrate—starch and sugar—but we'll get to that in detail in the next chapter.) To start with, the "milk shake" mix contains added fat. Regular mayonnaise and standard salad dressing contain significantly more fat than the "lite" or "lo-cal" products. The apple turnover contains oil in the pastry shell and is also fried in oil. The ice cream contains about 12 percent (more or less) fat.

That brings up another fringe benefit of the Quick Weight-Gain Program. You'll save money! Simply by avoiding foods that are labeled "lite," "lo-cal," "dietetic," "controlled calories," and all the other price-inflating adjectives, your food costs should go down as your weight goes up.

But don't worry—you won't have to do the job yourself. There are plenty of specific food suggestions, complete menus, and exciting recipes in the chapters that follow. The only thing we want to emphasize here is "fat awareness." When you are choosing your foods, think about the fat content. Always buy U.S. Choice beef if you can. It can have up to 6 percent more fat than the next lower priced grade in exactly the same cut.

When you make a sandwich, be sure not to trim the fat from the meat. Leave a generous border of fat around what you eat. When you are choosing a cut of meat, choose the one that has plenty of fat. Strangely enough, meat with a generous allotment of fat is more likely to come from a healthy animal. Think about it. That point was brought home to me in a most charming way some years ago in one of those delightful neighborhood open-air markets in Paris. It was a balmy spring morning, and I was picking up some roast beef for picnic sandwiches at noon. I pointed to a nice lean section of roast, and the wise old meatman shook his head.

''No, monsieur. That meat has no fat at all. That came from an emaciated animal who was too sick to put on weight. This one here''—and he pointed to a rosy side of beef flecked with marble-white fat—''this animal here was happy and healthy. It ate well and was able to gain some weight.''

It makes sense if you think about it. Oh yes, I know. Whenever we start talking about meat and fat, those creeping doubts come back. Don't all the magazines say that if you eat animal fat and ice cream and meat, you'll get all that terrible cholesterol clogging your arteries like so much grease in the drain of your kitchen sink? Well, stop worrying. First, your arteries aren't household plumbing. Secondly, *if* fat has anything to do with cholesterol deposits, it takes about 48 years or more to have an effect. Our goal is to put on about 1 pound a week. If you want to gain 10 pounds, that puts you on the Quick Weight-Gain Program for 10 weeks, not 48 years. Increasing your fat intake for a few months out of 80 years or so of a lifetime isn't going to do a normal person any harm.

And remember, as we have seen in chapter 2, being underweight is a greater risk to your health and life expectancy than eating the little bit of fat that will help you reach a healthy weight.

Okay, back to our job at hand—gaining weight quickly and easily. When you select a steak or chops at the market, don't let the butcher trim the fat away. You are handing him your weight gain instead of taking it home with you. Eat the meat, and eat the fat as well. Here's why:

Rescue those wasted calories to put on extra weight! Take a typical 1-pound well-trimmed (''well-trimmed'' really means that most of the fat is left on the butcher's cutting block) T-bone steak. It looks like a lot of protein, doesn't it? Let's look a little closer. There are about 1,850 calories in that steak.* Of those only about 420 calories are protein. The other 1,430 calories are fat. (There is no carbohydrate in beef.) If you just have the butcher leave 20 percent more fat around that steak, it will give you another 286

---

* All values are approximate due to individual differences in animals and calculations.

calories. Get him to leave 40 percent more fat and you'll be able to add 572 calories to your steak dinner. Just leaving 20 percent more fat on your steak dinner would add that extra pound in less than two weeks. At 40 percent more fat you'll have the extra pound on in less than a week. Of course you don't eat T-bone steak every night. (Do you?) But if we apply the same idea of rescuing wasted calories to everything we eat, the pounds will go on before we know it.

We can also pump up the calories by putting ketchup on our steak—4½ tablespoons will give us another 100 calories. Is it worth it? Sure it is. It's no extra effort to eat the ketchup—we'll hardly notice it. But that extra 100 calories will be in there working for us. If we prefer a gourmet touch instead, a mere half cup of buttery béarnaise sauce (bottled or canned) on top of that sizzling T-bone will give us another 175 calories or so. Over a period of time, twenty helpings of tasty béarnaise sauce translate into 1 extra pound of weight—nothing to be sneezed at.

The basic idea is this: Take advantage of any and every opportunity to add fat to your diet. Read the label on every food item before you buy it and look for the fat content. The more fat it has, the faster it will help you reach your goal.

In our battle against underweight we have two major weapons—two arrows in our quiver, so to speak. One of those arrows is fat—an effective and powerful means to restore the weight we need so badly. The other weapon is carbohydrate—starches and sugars. But carbohydrate is different. There are only some carbohydrates that are going to be helpful—and some can slow us down in our progress. In chapter 4 we'll find out which are allies and which are enemies. We'll also discover some exciting ways to combine carbohydrates with fats to make the combination much more effective than each individual component by itself. Chapter 4 is going to be a fascinating chapter. To get started, read on.

## Chapter Four

# Carbohydrates: Pick Them Right to Put on Pounds

**G**len just sat there shaking his head. Each time he shook it, he said the same word: "No, No, No."

"No what, Glen?"

"No way, Doctor! There's no way for me to gain weight! I've been trying to put on weight for the past six months and I'm thinner now than when I started!"

"How much do you weigh today, Glen?"

"One-twenty-two—and I'm 5 feet 10. And I'm 26 years old."

"Hmmm. That gives you a BMI of 17.5. And how much did you weigh before you began trying to put on weight?"

"One-twenty-five! And I've been eating like a pig! Sometimes I'm so full I feel like I'm going to burst. And it's October and I just have to put on some weight—fast!"

"That's interesting. What does October have to do with gaining weight, Glen?"

"It's a matter of my future, Doctor. I'm the Recreation Director at a big resort complex in Hawaii. Our season really gets underway toward the end of November. And you can imagine that I have to spend most of the day around the swimming pool or on the beach. We're playing volleyball, doing aerobics, playing active games, and generally jumping around. As you can imagine the Hawaiian beaches are full of muscular bodybuilder types—well developed, to say the least."

Glen paused a moment to pull up his shirt.

"Who can believe in a Recreation Director so skinny you can count his ribs. Look, there they are: one, two, three, four . . ."

"Okay, Glen, I'm convinced. But what have you been eating on your diet?"

"I got it out of one of those weight-lifting magazines that I bought at a newsstand. Now that I think about it maybe that wasn't exactly the most authoritative source. Well, anyhow, the article said if you want to gain weight, eat carbohydrates, and plenty of them. So I've been eating carbohydrates until they come out of my ears."

"What exactly have you been eating?"

"Well, I know all about fiber in food and how important it is so I've been careful to only eat carbohydrate with the highest fiber content. You know, I eat stone-ground 100 percent whole wheat bread, I eat organic pasta made from whole wheat with extra bran and wheat germ. I only eat brown rice—but the darkest I can find. And I eat about ¾ of a cup of bran a day besides. But after one plate of whole wheat spaghetti or macaroni, I'm so stuffed I can hardly move!"

"I'm not surprised. Your diet is excellent—"

Glen interrupted excitedly. "Excellent? Excellent? But if it's so *excellent,* how come I'm losing weight?"

"It's okay, Glen, take it easy. What I was saying was that your diet is excellent for someone who wants to *lose* weight. I certainly have to congratulate you for your dedication and hard work. But you only had half the puzzle. The high-fiber diet is a wonderful diet. It can accomplish a lot of things—but it just can't help you put on weight!"

"Are you sure, Doctor?"

"I'm sure, Glen. It so happens that I wrote the first book about the high-fiber diet. It was called *The Save-Your-Life Diet*[1] and it was published in 1975, long before anybody had even heard the name 'high-fiber.' It's a diet specifically designed to cut down on the absorption of calories, fill you up fast so you simply can't eat very much, and generally hold down your consumption of food. It also lowers cholesterol and prevents things like heart attacks and strokes.

"The high-fiber diet is an exceptionally healthy diet but *it won't help you with your current problem*. Remember that underweight is far more dangerous than cholesterol or overweight. Just like a low-fat diet, a high-fiber diet will protect you over the long term—say, your 80 years of life expectancy. But if you are really underweight, your chances of ever seeing that eightieth birthday are mighty slim.

"Glen, our immediate goal is to build up your weight to the point where you're healthy and at the same time make it hard for the girls on the beach to count your ribs. Then—and only then—can you start thinking about low fat and high fiber. Six months or so on a low-fiber, high-fat diet should be more than enough to restore you to normal weight—and all the benefits that go with it. Then you can spend the next 54 years on a low-fat, high-fiber diet if you wish. Our main goal is to put on pounds. Once you reach your normal weight we can pick the exact diet that will keep you permanently healthy—and happy."

The mistake that Glen made—and it wasn't his fault—was eating high-fiber carbohydrates. The fiber in those kind of carbohydrates actually functions as a wall against weight gain. No matter how much high-fiber carbohydrate you eat, you constantly bump up against the wall of fiber. Fiber makes the food that contains it harder to chew—and you eat less in the same period of time. Then it swells in your stomach when it's mixed with liquid and fills you up fast. Then it slows down the absorption of calories from the rest of your food as much as 20 percent. That means you can struggle to put away 3,000 calories but you'll only get the benefit of a mere 2,400. Simply put, a high-fiber diet gives you the exact *opposite* of what you want on a weight-gain program.

Now let's see how we can utilize carbohydrates to get exactly what we want from our weight-gain program. As we've seen, carbohydrates are the third in the group of basic food components, along with protein and fats. Actually there are two types of carbohydrate—and both of them are going to be very important to us in helping us achieve our goal. Let's take a moment to see what carbohydrates really are.[2] And we're going to get some surprises along the way.

The secret to understanding how to use carbohydrates to gain weight lies in one single word: *sugar*. That's because there are only two types of carbohydrates, both of them composed of sugar. One is called "starch" and consists of a kind of necklace of sugar molecules strung together like a string of pearls. The other type of carbohydrate is just plain sugar.

Before the starch form of carbohydrate can be used by our bodies it has to be converted to a simple form of sugar. When we eat a starchy food—like a piece of bread or a potato—digestion starts in the mouth and continues in the small intestine where the long strands of sugar are broken down into shorter strands. Among these short strands are a kind of complex sugar known as "maltose."*

In addition to sugars hooked together to form starch, we also eat several kinds of pure sugar in our daily diet. We eat "sucrose" in table sugar and "fructose" in honey, corn syrup, and soft drinks. Those are rarely a problem for us on our Quick Weight-Gain Program. But there is one other type of sugar that can be a stumbling block for certain of us.

Its name is "lactose," and it is found in milk and many (but not all) dairy products. It can sabotage our best efforts in the most unexpected manner. But there's a way around it, and we'll learn how to protect ourselves in chapter 11.

Specialized enzymes quickly digest all these sugars and convert them into substances we can use immediately for the needs of our bodies. That's a very important point. Our bodies can't utilize fried chicken or ice cream or string beans. All these very complicated foods have to be reduced to the one basic substance that our daily functioning depends on. That vital final product is "glucose," or the most common simple sugar that is found in our blood. Once the

---

* Actually these strands consist of maltose and isomaltose, but this step, like certain other technical details, has been simplified in this book.

starch we eat has been digested and converted to glucose, things suddenly get very interesting.

Our body weight, our strength and energy, and really our very survival, depend on what happens to that glucose. Once that sugar comes out of the digestive system and is poured into our blood it can go four different ways.[3] Which way it goes is very important for us and especially for those of us who want to gain weight. Some of the things that happen to that sugar are totally beyond our control. But some are not. And we need to learn how to control the ones that we can control.

The first possible destination for glucose once it gets into our blood is the liver, where it is stored as "glycogen." We want as much glucose as possible to go there as soon as possible to fill the liver with glucose in the form of glycogen so the liver won't absorb any more. Once the liver can't take any more glucose, the rest of the glucose is available to be stored as extra pounds!

The glucose that has escaped the clutches of the liver can still be trapped by the muscles and used for moving around—walking, running, riding a bike, or playing tennis. To gain weight, we want to minimize that activity so the sugar can go where we want it to go—into extra weight. So, as we noted before, we should avoid exercise after meals as much as possible.

A certain amount of glucose has to remain circulating in our bloodstream to supply our moment-to-moment needs. For example, the brain lives on glucose and needs a constant supply at all times. But any other glucose that isn't immediately needed goes right to— fat! That means extra weight for us—and fast!

That's why it is vitally important to keep our consumption of starch and sugar as high as possible. If we don't, our goal of putting on weight will recede farther and farther into the distance. If we don't eat enough carbohydrate, we might even bring on the disaster of "gluconeogenesis."[4] It's a big word and a bad word for anyone who is underweight—and it's a danger if we don't watch ourselves. If we don't consume enough carbohydrate every day to generously supply our body's needs, in desperation the protein that makes up our organs and muscles melts away and is converted by our bodies to the glucose we so badly need.

That's what that word means: "gluco" means "glucose," "neo" means "new," and "genesis" means "make." So *gluco-neo-genesis* means "make-new-glucose" but it also means "make it by eating away our organs and muscles!" That's one of the reasons why some people who are underweight are so underdeveloped and devoid of muscular strength. On the Quick Weight-Gain Program we'll make sure it doesn't happen but it's been bad news for more than one underweight person.

Now let's get to the question of how to strip away that wall of fiber that keeps us from getting the benefit of so many carbohydrates. (We should mention that you can look forward to complete, detailed menu plans in chapters 14 and 15—what follows are some interesting examples to get you started.)

Here's our basic problem: there are only 24 hours in a day. We can only eat so many times in that period, and we can only eat so much each time. In the meantime, our bodies are burning up calories minute by minute. Remember, it takes 1.5 calories a minute just to keep our bodies operating.[5] And if you're doing light office work or light housekeeping, you're eating up at least twice as many calories per hour. (That adds up to 180 calories per hour!) By the time you're 3,500 calories behind, you've lost another pound—another pound that you really can't afford to lose.

So, every bite at every meal has to count in order to get the maximum amount of calories into our bodies in the minimum amount of time. Fats play an important role in delivering a lot of calories in a small package. But as we have seen, fats have that satiety factor that kills our appetites so we can't eat as much of them as we might wish. But carbohydrate is different. If we do it right, we can eat a lot of carbohydrate before we get too full to continue. And since the average person eats up to 20 ounces of carbohydrate a day, that gives us plenty of opportunity to pick the highest calorie-carbohydrate combinations possible. That 20 ounces is usually divided between 12 ounces of starch, 6 ounces of table sugar, and about 2 ounces of lactose from milk products.

Remember that experience at the supermarket that we all have from time to time? We buy, let's say, a frozen cake. When we get it home, we have to rip open the clear plastic bag that it comes in. Then there's a cardboard box that we have to tear open. Then we get to that little aluminum foil cake pan and we have to pull off the cardboard top. Now we can see the cake, but we have to strip away one last layer of clear plastic covering before we can use it. By then we're so exhausted we can't really enjoy it. That's what they mean when they complain about "overpackaging."

Well, high-fiber carbohydrates are a perfect example of "overpackaging." Carbohydrates that have a lot of fiber are almost as hard for our bodies to process as it is us to open that armor-plated frozen cake. By the time we strip off the fiber and get down to the bare calories of the "complex" or high-fiber carbohydrate, there's not much left.

If we're ever going to put on that weight, what we need is a kind of carbohydrate where all the work has been done for us. That means we want *simple* or *low-fiber* carbohydrate. People who are trying hard to *lose* weight complain about food with "empty calories." But that's not really accurate for us. What we want is "unwrapped calories." We want calories without all that fiber that stands between us and the weight we want to put on. We'll get plenty of vitamins and minerals and protein from the Quick Weight-Gain Program. But we'll also get the calories we so desperately need.

So what we need on our diet is "simple" starches and sugar. Oh yes, I know what your friends are going to say: "Sugar? What about your teeth?" Well, sugar will only damage your teeth if you let it. If you allow residues of sugar or starch to remain in your mouth after you eat, they will ferment and decompose and form chemicals and bacteria that gradually attack your tooth enamel. Then the bacterial and chemical action continues, and your teeth start to decay. The solution? You'll find it right on the end of your toothbrush. Just brush your teeth after every meal—and if you can't brush for some reason, rinse your mouth thoroughly. But if it's a choice between a cavity (and it's not a choice, much less a danger, if you simply brush your teeth) and the 2,000-percent greater risk of death that underweight brings, I'll risk the cavity.

So we're going to look for "unwrapped" calories. That means enriched white flour, white flour pasta, white rice, and white bread. (Yes, that sinfully good cottony sliced white bread that made such wonderful peanut butter and jelly sandwiches is back on our diet—at least for the six months or so that we're going to dedicate to gaining weight.) We can sum up our carbohydrate philosophy this way: "If it's white, it's right!"

The proof is right there before us. A one-pound loaf of commercial whole wheat bread gives us about 1,100 calories. But a 1-pound loaf of commercial white bread has at least a hundred calories more. That's 66.6 minutes of extra fuel that can go toward building weight. And we get those extra calories free. We don't have to eat one bite more—we just have to consume the same pound of bread and at the same price—or less. So every 35 loaves of white bread gives us enough "free" extra calories for another pound of weight.

As we go through the menus in chapters 14 and 15 we'll see the tremendous advantage that our "simple carbohydrate" diet gives us. We'll find that just like the example of the white bread, we can eat exactly the same amount and yet get more calories to the bite. And even when the caloric values of the high-fiber starches are about the same as the low-fiber version, we'll be amazed at how much more low-fiber starch we can eat. For example, a plateful of high-fiber spaghetti is a meal in itself. It not only loads you up with the pasta—it saddles you with a lot of wrapping material in the form of fiber. That fiber fills you up but it won't put on an extra ounce.

On the other hand, good old white flour spaghetti slides down with no trouble. You'll be delighted at how much of it you can put away. And look at this example of the calories it can carry along with it:

Take 1 cup of spaghetti—and never cook it more than 10 minutes! Why? Because you'll cook the calories away! A cup of spaghetti cooked 10 minutes has 206 calories. Cook it for 20 minutes and you are left with a mere 150 calories. Without wanting to, you have boiled some of the starch out of the pasta and lost precious calories. Then add a 6-ounce jar of spaghetti sauce with meat at 270 calories. Top it off with ½ ounce of grated Parmesan cheese at 50 calories. For good measure you can also add 2 tablespoons of olive oil, which will give you another 250 calories extra. That gives you 776 calories for a mere cupful of spaghetti. It shouldn't be hard—depending on the circumstances—to even eat 2 cupfuls, which gives you 1,552 calories—just like that!

You can even come out ahead on something as simple as tortillas. A corn tortilla will give you about 70 calories while a wheat flour tortilla of the same size and weight gives you 5 calories more at 75 calories. Is it worth it? Sure it is. Look at the example of our overweight friends who don't even put a teaspoonful of sugar in their coffee. Every calorie counts—especially when you're burning them up every single minute of the day and night. If you want to gain weight, you must become a "calorie scavenger." Think of yourself as a calorie detective searching out every possible hidden calorie in every corner of your refrigerator or your kitchen cabinet and in every item on the menu in every restaurant where you eat.

Look at the tortilla example. If you eat 5 tortillas at a meal—not impossible—and you substitute wheat tortillas for corn tortillas, you will add 25 calories. That will replace almost 17 minutes of calories that you burn away every day. And the beauty of this method is that *you don't have to eat one bite more to get those extra calories.*

You can do the same thing when it comes to sugar. Remember that just like fats and carbohydrates, every bit of sugar that you don't need for energy goes right into extra weight. Except that sugar has one special advantage. Starch has to be digested—that is, processed by the body before it can be utilized as sugar.[6] That takes energy and uses up calories that we can't really spare. Those calories are better off going to add extra pounds. But sugar is already in the form where it can be used with little or no extra processing. Thus little or no extra calories have to be wasted digesting sugar.

We can get the same "free ride" with sugar that we got with starch if we know where to look. By consuming exactly the same amount of food or drink we can get extra calories without getting stuffed if we know where to look. Here are some examples:

The average person consumes about 2 quarts of liquid a day, more or less. For those of us who want to gain weight that opens up a wonderful opportunity that we want to take advantage of. The first principle is not to drink any *water* if you can help it—drink *liquid*. What's the difference between "liquid" and "water"? Well, liquid is water but with something else added. The caloric value of water is 0—yet it takes up as much space in your stomach as calorie-carrying liquid and gives you the same feeling of fullness. And you can only drink so much of it in a day. (Although you may not drink water be sure to get at least 8 glasses of *liquid* every 24 hours—and a little more won't hurt. But ideally every drop of that liquid should carry calories. If you prefer to drink some water, at least try to make the bulk of your fluid intake the kind that adds calories to your diet.) But if you manage to substitute 2 quarts of calorie-containing liquid for 0-calorie water, you'll be way ahead in your weight-gain program.

What kinds of calorie-containing liquid? Almost anything that is high in carbohydrates and high in calories—with certain exceptions that we'll see in a moment. Fruit drinks, milk-based drinks, soft drinks—there's a long list of possibilities.

How much good can these kinds of drinks do you? A lot of good. You'll be delighted when you see the figures. Let's take fruit drinks, for example. If you drink the canned or bottled so-called fruit punches or ades, you can expect to get as much as 140 calories per 8-ounce glass. If you drink 2 quarts of liquid a day, that adds up to 8 glasses of fruit punch or 1,120 extra calories that you wouldn't have gotten if you stuck to plain water. Now, most people aren't going to want 64 ounces of fruit punch a day. But if you only drink 2 glasses that's 280 calories that you wouldn't get otherwise. You've managed to put back 3 hours and 11 minutes of calories that you burned by just living and cleared the way for adding those badly needed pounds. And all you did was drink the liquid that you were going to drink anyway! If you prefer fruit juices, freshly squeezed orange juice will give you 110 calories extra. (The punches go down easier because they contain a higher percentage of water, of course.)

What you are getting in prepared fruit drinks basically is a good dose of carbohydrates—no fat, no protein. They consist of fruit juice, added sugar, and water. It's not nutritional perfection, but it doesn't have to be. What we want right now is calories in abundance in a way that goes down easy.

There are many opportunities in the world of soda as well. You can drink whatever is around or you can be a calorie detective, ferreting out the best possible source of calories in the smallest possible bite—or sip. For example, you can drink ginger ale at 80 calories per 8-ounce glass. But for the same amount of liquid, you can sip cherry pop or cream soda at about 130 calories! That 50 calories per glass will counterbalance more than half an hour of your minute-by-minute calorie burn-off. Your best bets for calories per ounce are the fruit-flavored sodas like orange, grape, and strawberry. But here's another tip. Most of the fruit-flavored carbonated drinks don't taste too awfully sweet—that's because of the large amount of fruit acid they contain. If you like, you can add up to a tablespoon of ordinary sugar to a glass. That gives you another 40 calories. Even if you only add a teaspoon of sugar, that's at least 13 calories more—or about 8½ minutes of what our bodies use up at rest. Every little bit counts—and it's *all* carbohydrate.

If you like chocolate, you're in luck. Both cocoa and chocolate-flavored instant mixes will give you about 115 calories in an 8-ounce glass if you use 3 teaspoons of the powder. But use more—after you make sure that what you're using contains added sugar. If you use 2 tablespoons, you can double the caloric value without really noticing a difference in taste. Add a tablespoon of whipping cream and you can get another 50 calories into the glass. With double powder and a little shot of cream your drink will be 280 calories. Not bad. You can get about the same with the premixed milk shakes or chocolate breakfast drinks from the supermarkets. Just read the label carefully to make sure you're getting the most calories for your efforts.

There's another drink that you just might like. In a sense it's a secret weapon against underweight. It's an interesting beverage that has come up from Latin America, where it is a real favorite. People have been underweight in that part of the world for decades—not so much because of poverty but because of the traditional diet. The usual Latin American diet is high fiber—full of fresh fruit and vegetables and high-fiber bread and tortillas. But underweight people there have relied on this unique beverage to help them put on the weight they need.

The general name for the drink is "Malta," which means, of course, *malt*. "Malta" is a fascinating hybrid drink best described as beer without alcohol enriched with extra natural sugars. Malta is not "near beer" and it is certainly not "malt liquor." (Malt liquor is an alcoholic drink like beer but with a higher alcohol content.) Malta has a rich sweet malty flavor and a minimum of 175 calories in each 8-ounce glass, substantially more than most soft drink or fruit punches and even higher than beer itself.

But Malta has a sort of "secret-weapon" quality. Since most high-carbohydrate drinks fill you up and satisfy your appetite, their effect is limited to adding weight. But beyond that, Malta, because of its nonalcoholic but beer-related ingredients, tends to actually stimulate the appetite. An hour or so after you drink a glass, you may find yourself eager to eat. That's the "secret weapon" part. You might be able to find it at any big supermarket—ask around. And be sure to drink it icy cold—that's the way everyone does in Latin countries. You just might like it. If you do, it will make you gain weight a little faster. If it's not exactly your taste, don't worry—we have plenty other weight-gaining tricks up our sleeve.

What about beer? Well, beer or any other alcoholic beverage is a two-edged sword. If you have one beer a day with your supper, it can add its calories without adding other problems. But if one beer leads to another, then you may end up displacing good solid calorie-containing foods. I know about the ''beer bellies'' on dedicated beer drinkers. But there are two things against that for people like us. First, we don't want a big potbelly. The idea is to gain weight sensibly and attractively. Secondly, those beer bellies are usually the result of years of dedicated consumption of beer. We don't want to wait years to put on those pounds. We want to accomplish our goal promptly—hopefully within six months or so. All in all, the best approach is this: if you already drink beer, you can continue provided it doesn't interfere with your consumption of high-calorie foods. But don't start to drink beer with the hope that it will help you. It's not necessary.

What about wine? Once again, a few ounces of wine before dinner can help us in our program. Some people find that wine stimulates their appetite and encourages them to eat more. Other folks find it makes them sleepy and disinterested in food. The best approach is the same as for beer. If you already drink wine, you can continue provided it doesn't interfere with your consumption of high-calorie foods. But don't start to drink wine with the hope that it will help you.

What about ''hard'' liquor—whiskey, rum, vodka, and all the rest? Exactly the same approach. A drink before dinner may help you, but don't start drinking distilled spirits to gain weight. It's not an essential part of the program.

There are two common everyday beverages that don't have any place on a weight-gaining diet. They are: tea and coffee. Both of them contain caffeine or caffeine-like chemicals and virtually no calories at all. Why work for nothing if you can do the same job and get paid for it? Why drink 8 ounces of liquid if you're not getting any calories for all the effort you're putting out? In the ten minutes it takes to sip a cup of tea or coffee, you're losing at least 15 calories and not getting anything back. In the same amount of time you could be sipping a nice fruit punch or a grape soda and get enough calories to put on some weight in the process. That brings us to the first two basic principles of weight gain:

1. There are only 24 hours in a day and your body burns up calories as each minute goes by—even if you don't even lift a pencil. If you use as many of those minutes as reasonably possible to absorb calories, you can gain weight. If you waste your time on foods that don't give you fair caloric value, you'll have a harder time gaining those pounds.

2. Each of us wakes up every morning with a certain limited "appetite potential." That is, we can only eat so much each day before we get "full" and can't eat another bite. If we squander our "appetite potential" on food and drinks that fill us without giving us the calories we need, we may never gain weight—and we can actually lose ounces day by day. So before you eat or drink, ask yourself this: "Is what I am about to consume going to help me reach my goal of putting on pounds?" If not, *don't eat it* but substitute something else that will add calories.

Now that we have seen how our second great ally—carbohydrates—can help us in our war against underweight, we are ready to put everything we have learned into practice. With all that we already know—plus what we are going to find out as we go along—we're going to have an easy and enjoyable time adding those extra pounds.

## Chapter Five

# Weight-Gain Strategy: The Key to Success

**N**ow comes the time to plan our strategy of weight gain. And the right word is "strategy." Just eating high-calorie foods isn't enough to do the job. If it were that easy, Suzanne would have solved her problem long ago.

Suzanne was pretty and blonde—29 years old and 5 feet 2 inches tall. She weighed 97 pounds. That gave her a Body Mass Index of 17.85, well under the minimum BMI of 19 to 20.[1] As it happened, her job as Director of Nursing at a large teaching hospital was a real physical and mental strain for someone that much underweight.

"Could it be possible, Doctor, for someone to be immune to food?"

"Immune to food? That's an interesting concept, Suzanne. What makes you ask?"

"Well, I think that's my problem. I eat and eat and eat and still I can't gain weight!"

"How do you select the food on your diet?"

Suzanne smiled.

"I use what I call the 'Jack Sprat' approach."

"Hmmm. How does that work?"

"Well, you remember the rhyme:

> Jack Sprat could eat no fat,
> His wife could eat no lean.

> And so betwixt the two of them,
> They licked the platter clean!

"I just watch my overweight friends and everything they don't dare eat, I gobble up. They wouldn't eat potato chips if their lives depended on it and I eat them by the bag. Chocolate cake? They don't even want to see chocolate cake. I eat two and three pieces at a time. Cookies? I love 'em! I eat half a dozen for dessert. But it's like all that fattening food doesn't have any effect on me. That's why I asked you—half-seriously—if I'm 'immune' to food."

"No, it's nothing like that, Suzanne. It's just a matter of planning. You can't gain weight by just doing the opposite of what people who want to lose weight are doing."

She wrinkled her pretty brow. "But why not?"

"Because being underweight is not simply the opposite of being overweight. People who are substantially overweight have a different metabolism because they have distorted the *way their body* works by putting on so many pounds.[2] That's why they can gain weight on potato chips and you can't. That's also the reason why so many amateur—and even professional—weight-gaining programs fail. Remember what we discovered about carbohydrates: fiber makes a big difference. Although potato chips are 40 percent fat, they are also 1.6 percent fiber. That means they have as much fiber as whole wheat bread! Besides, they are loaded with salt. [And the salt probably has added iodine. A few pages farther on, we'll see how that iodine can sabotage you.]

"The fiber fills you up fast, the salt makes you thirsty and when you drink loads of water, guess what happens? That 1.6 percent fiber soaks up the water, swells in your stomach, and you're all through eating for quite awhile. But overweight people, on the other hand, love that feeling of fullness and often it even motivates them to eat more. When you feel full, you're finished eating. When they get full, they're just getting started."

"But what about the chocolate cake I eat—with chocolate frosting?"

"Was it a devil's food cake?"

"Yes! The most fattening!"

"Let's see how fattening it really was. The usual devil's food cake with chocolate frosting is about 370 calories in the average 3½-ounce serving. That sounds good but . . ."

Suzanne threw up her hands. "Now don't tell me, Doctor, that chocolate cake isn't fattening!"

"Sure, it is. But 'fattening' isn't enough. For a food item to help us gain weight it has to be loaded with calories—that's vital. But it also has to be in a form that we can eat enough of to do us good. And it has to be in a form that will allow us to keep eating more of it and other fattening foods besides."

"And chocolate cake doesn't fill the bill?"

"Let's take a look. Devil's food cake with chocolate frosting is 55 percent carbohydrate and only 16 percent fat. That means you have to eat your way through a lot of carbohydrate with only 4.1 calories per gram before you get the benefit of the 6 percent fat. That 6 percent fat offers you more than twice as many calories per gram—9.3 to be exact. The problem is, you get filled up on the carbohydrate long before the fat can do you much good."

Suzanne's eyes widened. "Then what's the solution?"

" 'WGS,' Suzanne. 'WGS.' Plain old 'Weight-Gain Strategy.' Just eat exactly the same amount of cake but substitute pound cake for devil's food. With chocolate frosting at about 120 calories, the same-size piece of old-fashioned pound cake will give you almost 600 calories. And it won't make you feel one bit fuller than that piece of devil's food. That pound cake is only 47 percent carbohydrate but a whopping 30 percent fat or almost twice the fat of the chocolate cake. So you eat exactly the same amount of food but you get nearly twice as many calories for your efforts—600 versus 370."

Suzanne nodded. "Very interesting, Doctor. But what about cookies? I eat plenty of cookies, and I know they're full of sugar and fat but they never seem to help me put on weight!"

"What kind of cookies do you eat, Suzanne?"

"Fig bars! I love fig bars! And I eat them all the time!"

"Fig bars are probably the perfect choice—for someone who loves cookies and needs to lose weight. The standard portion—say 3½ ounces of fig bars—only gives you 358 calories. That's bad enough but it also loads you up with a hefty 1.7 percent of fiber. That's twice as much fiber as brown rice! If you're looking for a cookie that will help you put on weight, try chocolate chip cookies. A standard recipe will give you 516 calories in the same 3½ ounces with less than ½ of 1 percent fiber. Remember, it's the same amount of cookie to eat but you're getting at least 30 percent more calories for the same effort. If you don't like chocolate chip cookies, you can substitute any of the dozens of those high-calorie cookies that line the supermarket shelves. They will give you plenty of calories easily and effectively."

By the way, most of those weight-gaining recipes in chapters 14 and 15 are "enhanced" recipes. That means they are all packed with extra calories that are "invisible." Those are calories that add pounds—but you won't even know they are there. And all these dishes are a pleasure to eat—they are loaded with taste appeal and flavor. The best part is that many of the enhanced recipes take hardly any effort at all. If you work or just don't have the inclination to do a lot of cooking, you can follow the simple instructions and really increase the calories of standard supermarket foods without any inconvenience.

Here's an example. Let's say you've chosen a high-calorie salad dressing from the list in chapter 12. It could be a brand of Italian dressing with 100 calories per tablespoon. You're going to put 4 tablespoons on your salad—that's 400 calories. Not bad. But what if you add a little extra olive oil to that bottle of dressing? If it's a 6-ounce bottle, just add about 1½ ounces of extra olive oil. The only difference you should notice is that it will make the dressing taste even better. But with no effort at all you've raised the caloric value about 25 percent.* That means you should get about 500 calories from those 4 tablespoons of Italian dressing. So without having to eat one more bite of food you are adding precious calories.

---

* All caloric values are approximate—but close enough to help you put on those pounds.

If you use the "enhanced salad dressing" every day (it doesn't have to be Italian—it could just as well be French dressing, Thousand Island, Green Goddess or whatever you like) you will soon see the results. In 35 days, if you don't do anything else to help yourself, you will see an extra pound or so on the scale. And of course, you're going to do a lot of other things to help yourself.

That's only one example. In chapter 15 you will find plenty more ways to add calories to everyday convenience foods. Besides that, if you like to cook for yourself or for someone who needs to gain weight, there is a wonderful collection of enhanced recipes you can make from scratch. They include everything from appetizers to desserts, and each and every one of them adds hundreds of extra invisible calories to each dish.

While we're on the subject of menu recommendations, there is one specific thing we can do right now today to advance our cause. Remember when we discussed the problem of metabolism and a thyroid gland that works too hard? If the thyroid is speeding up our metabolism, we'll have trouble putting on weight, no matter how much we eat. One of the things we can do is slow down our thyroid just enough to make our weight gain that much more efficient. The safest and simplest way to do that is simply to apply what we have learned. Remember, the thyroid needs a constant supply of iodine in our diet to make the thyroid hormones. If we make that iodine harder to find, then there wouldn't be so much hormone available. But how can we lock up some of that iodine?

Fortunately there's a safe and easy way to do it. Certain common foods "trap" the iodine in our diet so that it can't be made into thyroid hormone. The effect is very gentle and, best of all, temporary. When we add these "iodine-trappers" to our diet, our thyroid should slow down a bit. As soon as we cut back on these foods, the thyroid immediately has more iodine available and can speed up our bodies' metabolism. (So over the long run we're not going to affect the function of our thyroid gland one bit.)

The effect is almost like magic. It's easy and appetizing to include these foods in our diet, and if it works for us, we can gain more weight faster and with much less effort. The only other thing we have to do to get the most benefit from this method of controlling our own metabolism is make sure not to consume too much iodine.

Unfortunately most of us get a big slug of iodine every day of our lives, whether we want to or not. This is one of the outdated left-overs from the medical practices of the last century that is still with us. It happened this way:

Many millions of years ago, during the last Ice Age, glaciers (gigantic rivers of ice) covered much of the northern United States. When these ice rivers finally receded as the climate changed and the temperature rose, they dragged with them part of the topsoil and some of the minerals it contained. Among the minerals that were depleted was—iodine!

In the United States during the 1800s, most people ate vegetables that were raised on farms within 50 miles or so of their homes. They were delivered by horse-drawn wagon, and of course there was no refrigeration. So if you lived in the Middle West, your food was grown in soil that was deficient in iodine. That meant that the food itself was deficient in iodine.

A serious clinical deficiency of iodine causes a compensating swelling of the thyroid gland as the gland enlarges to try to do more with less. That enlargement is called a "goiter," and the area of the country where soil was deficient in iodine was known as the "Goiter Belt." The experts of that time decided, wisely, that the people needed more iodine in their diet. Since the people of that era were generally poorly informed and unsophisticated medically, they couldn't be trusted to take iodine pills and much less give them to their children. So the experts decided to add iodine to the salt! The reasoning was simple: everyone ate salt so everyone would get their dose of iodine that way without even knowing it. It worked, and the goiters almost disappeared.

But that was 1800! And this is today! With refrigeration and fast-freezing and modern transportation everyone gets food from all over the country, if not the world. There is plenty of iodine in everyone's diet—they don't need the experts to give them an extra slug of the chemical in their salt.

To make matters worse, iodine isn't that good for you. It makes acne and other skin conditions worse, it can trigger thyroid problems in susceptible persons, and it's in your salt whether you want it or not. Most important of all, it's in your salt in therapeutic doses—that is, there's enough of it in your salt to act as a medicine. If you need iodine your doctor will give you a prescription. You don't have to have it forced on you without your permission. Most important of all, it can sabotage your attempts to gain weight by flooding your thyroid with too much iodine and thereby raising your metabolic rate.

So, for this very effective and useful technique to work you have to be sure to stay away from extra iodine. Luckily, it's not too hard. Don't use iodized salt—you can identify it since it has to be marked on the label. Don't eat food made with seaweed. Seaweed? Does that sound funny? Well, not anymore. With Oriental food now fashionable you get more seaweed than you imagine. Many of the soups and broths contain seaweed, sushi is wrapped in seaweed, and many other dishes contain it. When you're dining Oriental, just keep your eyes open—and ask if you're not sure.

To keep your thyroid from turning up your thermostat and burning away those hard-won calories, make sure you include at least one serving of iodine-trapping foods every day in your diet. These are members of the Cruciferae family and they have the special ability to keep excess iodine from getting to the thyroid where it can work against you. Ideally they should be eaten raw—cooking keeps them from grabbing the iodine. Here they are:

broccoli
cauliflower
cabbage
Chinese cabbage
cress
mustard

peppergrass
radish
roquette

Obviously the best way to eat these iodine-hunters raw is in salads. With that in mind you'll find some hints for some high-calorie anti-iodine salad recipes in chapter 15. You'll be amazed and delighted at the variety and the appeal of these very useful and important weapons in our campaign to gain weight.

You should also be sure to include nuts in your daily diet. They can be walnuts, almonds, pecans, pistachios, cashews, or macadamias. In addition to adding needed calories, many of them also trap iodine and aid in slowing fast metabolism. By the way, that doesn't include peanuts, which as you know are not nuts at all but really a sort of bean. However, peanuts play a very important and useful role in our weight-gain program, as we'll see later on. You'll find them all included in a whole gamut of recipes in chapters 14 and 15.

As they start to put weight on, there is one question that occurs to almost every one of my patients. Nancy put it this way:

"I'm really happy to put on weight, Doctor, especially after all these years of suffering. And it has been suffering. Who likes to buy A-cup brassieres and clothes that don't really fit? And when a man puts his arms around me and feels nothing but bones? They don't always say something but occasionally they make remarks like, 'Have you been sick lately or something?' I mean, it's not exactly what a girl looks forward to. Especially at the ripe old age of 26. I mean, now that I'm filling out, I'm looking forward to a lot more fun. But there is one thing that bothers me."

"What's that, Nancy?"

"Well, I've put on 5 pounds so far in a little over a month. I can see the difference in my bra size. I'm a B cup for the first time in my life and it feels great! I also see a little fullness in my hips—like my panties are starting to feel tight. But I don't want to get a big fat belly and a big rear end! How do we control that? Or can we control it?"

"It doesn't have to be a problem. In women, because of the influence of female sex hormones—basically estrogen—the weight you gain goes to specific places.[3] You described it correctly—to the breasts and the hips. Those are storage points for the energy needs of future pregnancies and milk production for your babies. Besides that, the fat you gain is an important secondary source of estrogen. Although not many people are aware of it, estrogen is synthesized in adipose tissue or fat. That's one of the reasons that women with ample fat deposits have an easier time in the menopause than very thin women."

Nancy smiled. "I'm glad to hear that!"

"I understand that you have a long way to go before you have to think about the menopause. But there's an immediate benefit waiting for you as soon as you start to put on weight. It's a kind of 'one-good-thing-leads-to-another' situation. As you begin to put on weight in the form of fat, that fat helps to synthesize more estrogen. That same estrogen encourages the development of your breasts and also feminizes your hips and buttocks. As it deposits more fat on the hips and in the breasts, that same adipose tissue produces more estrogen.

"But the good news doesn't stop there. Your increased production of estrogen makes it easier for you to gain weight. It also keeps your ovaries, uterus, and vaginal tissues in tip-top condition. It also gives you wonderfully effective protection against heart attacks."[4]

"But, Doctor, I've read that too much estrogen can be bad for you."

"That's a controversial topic in medicine these days, and doctors don't agree among themselves. But the controversy is about exogenous estrogen—the kind you take in pills or injections like birth control pills and that sort of thing. Your own body makes endogenous estrogen—that's totally natural and completely harmless to you. There's no controversy about that. So as you add fat, you make yourself more feminine at the same time your own increased estrogen makes it even easier to continue gaining weight."

Nancy sighed.

"Well, that's a relief!"

"Certainly. But getting back to your question about controlling the amount of weight we gain. It's not really going to be a problem. There's good news there, too. Since we're putting on the weight slowly—a pound or so at a time—we can keep track of exactly where it's going and where we want it to go. Keep your tape measure handy and measure your hips and your breasts—and your waist. And of course, calculate your Body Mass Index about once a week. Once your Body Mass Index gets up to between 22 and 24 you have reached a reasonable weight goal. And now, Nancy, would you mind if I guessed what your next question is going to be?"

She chuckled good-naturedly. "Go right ahead, Doctor."

"You're going to ask, 'But what if I add enough weight to my breasts but my hips are still too small?' or 'What if I add enough weight to my hips but my breasts are still too small?' "

Nancy nodded her head slowly. "I get the feeling that you've been through this before."

"Only about a thousand times. There are two answers to that kind of question. First, the Quick Weight-Gain Program can't guarantee you a perfect body because there is no such thing as a 'perfect body.' The human body is designed to function as a complex living organism, not to win beauty contests or be trotted out in fashion shows. But adding weight will certainly improve your appearance at the same time it improves your health and vitality.

"Secondly, you can control the way the weight goes to a great extent. Of course the size of your breasts is determined primarily by genes. If your mother and grandmother had small breasts, you are not likely to get to a 38-D. But you will certainly increase the size and attractiveness of your breasts as you add pounds.

"The same concepts apply to your hips. On the Quick Weight-Gain Program you will add curves to straight hips as you deposit fat. That's why women look like women—because of the subcutaneous fat deposits that give roundness to their bodies. But where to stop? That's a matter of personal taste. Most women like round hips and round buttocks—to fill out their clothes in an appealing way. But most of them prefer to draw the line at fat hips and fat buttocks. But you can control it. Watch your mirror, watch your tape measure, feel how your clothes fit, and switch to the Hold-Your-Weight Diet when you want to stop gaining but you don't want to lose pounds.''

Nancy broke in. ''But isn't there anything else I can do?''

''Sure there is. You can 'mold' that weight that you are putting on. You can make it more prominent in just the areas that you want to emphasize.''

''Like my breasts, for example?''

''Like your breasts. Exactly. When your hips are as well developed as you want them to be, but your breasts are not quite as large as you want them, you can stop gaining weight. Then you can 'mold' your breasts—within limits of course—to make them seem larger in proportion to your hips.''

Her eyebrows went up. ''And how can I accomplish that?''

''By doing some very simple exercises. Behind both breasts, Nancy, on the chest wall, there are several sets of muscles. If you develop those muscles, they enlarge and push the breasts up and out. They make them seem larger or, better put, the breasts actually become larger in the sense that you will need a larger size brassiere. And they raise the breasts higher at the same time.''

''But that's a lot of weight lifting and all that, isn't it?''

''No, it's not very hard at all. The muscles are active in everyday movements and it's fairly simple to develop them and enlarge them. If you put in 10 minutes a day you should see satisfying results in about a week.''

''Wow! Where do I get those exercises?''

''They're all in chapter 5. But since you asked, here's a sample of the kind of exercise that will help to 'mold' your breasts. But remember, they won't make your breast tissue firmer. That's made up of fat and glandular tissue. But they will enlarge the muscles behind your breasts and push the breasts upward and outward. If you do the exercises regularly and stay with your weight-gain program it should only be a matter of time before you're wearing the next-size bra cup.''

Nancy leaned forward, just a little. "What are the exercises like? How do I do them?"

"First, you have to assemble the equipment."

"Equipment? I need equipment?"

"Well, you could call it that. Do you have a piece of broomstick or a length of bamboo about 2 feet long around the house?"

"Of course!"

"How about a footstool or a hassock about 15 inches high, more or less?"

"Sure."

"You're in luck, Nancy! That's all the equipment you need. Here are 2 excellent exercises—you'll find them simple to do.

"Sit down on the footstool with your feet on the floor about 2 feet apart. Hold the piece of broomstick with one hand at each end straight above your head. Then lean forward as if you were going to put your head on your knees. At the same time lower the broomstick so that it's behind your head at the back of your neck. The final position should be leaning way over with your head almost on your knees and the broomstick held at the back of your neck. Then straighten up so that the broomstick is up in the air above your head like before, and you're sitting just like when you started."

"It sounds easy."

"It is easy, but if we understand the medical and scientific principles behind what we do, it doesn't have to be hard. Do that exercise about 5 times or so the first day and after a while you should be able to gradually raise it to about 25 times a day. Don't force it. Just do what you can do comfortably. You will feel the difference in a day or so, and you'll see the difference in about two weeks."

"What's the next exercise? You said there were two."

"I have at least 15 that I can recommend but these two are the easiest and the most effective. Here's the second one and it's really sensational. Don't overdo it—it looks simple but it will build up those pectoral muscles faster than you can imagine. Here goes.

"Sit down on the same footstool. Hold the broomstick behind your back at waist level. Sit up straight and slowly raise both arms upward until the broomstick is about level with your shoulders. Hold that position for the count of 3 and then bring your arms down slowly.

"Repeat it about 5 times. If you get tired, let it go until the next day. Gradually work it up until you are holding the broomstick up for 6 seconds each time and doing about 15 repetitions. But don't force it. Just do it gradually. After 2 weeks or so you can advance to the next stage if you really want those breasts to be more prominent. Instead of a broomstick, hold a can of soup in each hand. That adds a little weight and makes the muscles enlarge even faster.

"I think you'll be amazed at how those muscles grow. If you want to feel the power of these deceptively simple exercises, do them with one hand while you hold the muscle that goes from your shoulder to your breast with the other. You can feel the muscle straining and bulging. 'Muscle molding' with the Quick Weight-Gain Program really works!

"And here is an excellent exercise for molding the lower hips and buttocks to enhance their shape, make them more compact, and reduce any tendency to flabbiness. By 'molding,' you can hold the effects of your weight gain back where you want to and increase it wherever it seems desirable. Here's an excellent exercise.

"This is ideal for shaping the hips and enlarging the gluteus muscles. These are the muscles that you sit on, and one of the problems with underweight is that the buttocks sometimes seem to almost disappear. This exercise will give you well-rounded but firm buttocks to fill out your best clothes without exaggerating any dimension. And it's simple and almost effortless—but amazingly effective.

"Kneel on a comfortable rug on all fours. Raise one knee off the ground about 4 inches. Then stretch your leg backward all the way as if you were trying to touch something behind and above you with your toe. Hold it there for a moment while you tighten the muscles in your buttocks. Then slowly bring the leg back to the original position. Do the same thing with the other leg—slowly and easily. Repeat it 3 times at first, gradually increasing as the days go by until you're doing about 10 a day. You will be amazed and delighted with the results.''

"But what about my husband? He's thin too, and he's going to start on the weight-gain diet. But is he going to have bigger breasts?"

"Hardly. Weight gain in men is also directed by hormones. That's why most of the adipose tissue in men is deposited in the abdominal area—right on the belly.[5] That's where it's available for quick energy on long hunting expeditions and other prehistoric tasks that most men don't do anymore. If a man finds that he is depositing fat on his breasts and hips, he should see his doctor right away. He may well have a hormone problem that needs to be looked into.''

"But then how does a man control his weight gain?"

"It's fairly easy. When his trousers start getting tight in the waist and when his tape measure tells him that his waist is expanding more than he wants it to, it's time to cut back on the calories. But he can take advantage of the same 'molding' techniques that women can use. Of course, the exercises are different. Here's an example:

"To define the waist and give bulk to the abdomen, this exercise is easy and effective. Lie down on the floor on your back—put a pillow under the small of your back extending up to just under your shoulders. Bend your knees at a comfortable angle—about 30 to 40 degrees. That takes any strain off your back. Clasp your hands behind your head and bend forward and upward until your elbows just touch your knees. Then lean back until your shoulders *almost* touch the floor but never go all the way down. Hold it there a moment and then sit up again. Start with 5 repetitions—no more. Gradually work up slowly day by day until you are doing 20 or so. Don't overdo it—there is no benefit to straining yourself. If you feel any pain or discomfort, stop immediately and consult your doctor, of course.''

Now that we have seen the benefits of fat in our diet and the benefits of carbohydrate in our diet, it's logical to ask a fascinating question: What happens if we combine both fats and carbohydrate in a single dish?

The answer is that, scientifically speaking, we should get exactly the same benefit as if we ate the two or more components separately. But in the real world it doesn't seem to work that way. For some reason that no one really understands, eating fats and carbohydrate together seems to give faster gains than eating them separately.

Now, no one can prove this either way but it's worth giving it a try in your menu planning. Here are a few typical fat-carbohydrate combinations that you can easily work into your diet, along with their caloric values. Try it, it can't hurt. Many patients have reported excellent gains with these combinations, and they just might work for you. In any event, you'll get the full caloric benefit either way.

One of my favorites is the ice-cream sundae. Look at what it offers:

1. Ice cream: fat in the form of butterfat (up to 14 percent or so) and carbohydrate in the form of sugar. 1 cup is about 350 calories.
2. Chocolate (or other flavor) syrup—some fat (if it's chocolate) with plenty of carbohydrate—up to 350 calories in 4 tablespoons.
3. Nuts in syrup—fat and carbohydrate—up to 350 calories in 4 tablespoons.
4. Whipped cream—fat and carbohydrate—one ounce at 55 calories.

So a simple chocolate (or other flavor) sundae offers you 1,105 calories plus the possible benefit of an added effect between fat and carbohydrate. Three of those will put you close to an extra pound of weight. Now, you can't eat ice-cream sundaes all day. But maybe you can slip one in at bedtime or in the middle of the afternoon. Even if you only manage one or two a week, you'll be doing a lot to advance your cause. And the nice thing about a sundae is that it just slides right down. Basically it is only liquid, except for the nuts.

If you're on the run and can't sit down for a sundae, a deluxe ice-cream cone is almost as good. If you get a double-decker chocolate-dipped with nuts and anything else you can think of, it should add up to about half the calories of a sundae, say 500 or so. Not bad for a snack on the run.

Another excellent combination is the old American standby: peanut butter and jelly sandwiches. They have everything to help you gain weight and in an appetizing package (if you like peanut butter and jelly, of course). Look at the way it adds up:

4 tablespoons of peanut butter—400 calories on the average.
4 tablespoons of jelly—200 calories.
2 slices of white bread—160 calories. Look for the highest calorie white bread, of course.

So a simple little peanut butter and jelly sandwich gives you a nice 760-calorie push toward your goal. And it shouldn't fill you up too much in the process.

But you have to be careful when you're combining fats and carbohydrates. For example, one ounce of peanuts gives us about 180 calories. That's not bad considering that peanuts are 20 percent carbohydrate and a respectable 48 percent fat. Now let's go one step further. Let's add a chocolate covering to the peanuts. That should give us the extra calories that we are always looking for.

Let's see. One ounce of chocolate-covered peanuts will give us a disappointing 150 calories. What happened? We've lost 30 calories in the deal! That's a 17 percent loss in calories. If you snack on chocolate-covered peanuts to add a few extra ounces as you go along, you will actually be losing out! You're eating as much, you're getting just as full, but you're not getting the same caloric value per ounce. What went wrong?

Just this. That chocolate covering is mostly sugar and it adds weight without really adding much in the way of calories. So an ounce of chocolate-covered peanuts has more coating but less peanuts by weight. These are just the kinds of things we are going to learn about as we go along.

That brings us to the next step. Now we're ready to get into some meal planning and sample menus so that we can put all our knowledge to work for us and begin to really gain weight.

## Chapter Six

# The Caloric Bill of Rights, CCK, OFD, and Other Tricks of the Trade

**Y**ou know, Doctor, I've spent hours and hours trying to analyze it and I just can't make any sense out of it.''

When Rick talked like that I knew something was up. He was 31 and one of the country's leading chemical engineers. He founded his own company when he was 19 and he was a millionaire many times over. He was also 6 feet tall, blond with piercing green eyes—and he weighed 131 pounds. That gave him a Body Mass Index of 17.8, or as he was happy to point out to me, 17.803942. But no matter where you rounded it off, he was significantly underweight. Now, if there was something that Rick couldn't analyze, it must be complicated.

"What is it, Rick, that puzzles you?"

He rubbed his chin and hesitated a moment.

"It's this, Doctor. I've been underweight all my life—at least as long as I can remember. I've been trying to find a solution on my own, and as you can see, I haven't had much success. I try to eat as much as I can but my biggest problem is I get full too soon. I mean, I get to the point where I just can't eat any more. I know I should be taking in more calories but I simply don't have room in my stomach.'' He stopped suddenly and put up his hand. "No! That's wrong! I know I have room in my stomach because I know the volume of what I have swallowed and I know the volume of my stomach. Mechanically, I'm not 'full,' but I feel like I can't eat another bite! What's the explanation?''

"You certainly have an analytical mind, Rick. You put your finger on a very important problem for everyone who is underweight. Even with excellent motivation and good discipline, so often patients find it difficult to eat enough. Just like you said, they get 'full' before the meal is over. And you were right about something else. That 'fullness' is a psychological feeling, not a physical one. The proof is there for anyone to see."

"For example, Doctor?"

"Well, overweight people sometimes take a pill containing something called 'carboxymethylcellulose,' a by-product of cotton. If you swallow a pill of carboxymethylcellulose and drink some water, the substance swells up in your stomach and fills it up. But it doesn't really satisfy you, and most important, it doesn't kill your hunger. So as you suspected from your own observations, you don't feel 'full' or satisfied just because your stomach is distended with food. But if we're going to really put on weight easily and effectively, we need to know why we get full and how to postpone that feeling of being stuffed as long as possible. If we can only put it off another 5 minutes or so at each meal, we have that much time to eat more calories before we have to stop."

"Sounds logical, Doctor. But what's the answer?"

"For a long time, nobody knew. But some years ago scientists began to study a mysterious hormone known as 'cholecystokinin,' or CCK for short.[1] Cholecystokinin is what we doctors call a 'neuropeptide.'[2] That's a substance formed during the process of digestion that acts on the nervous system to produce an effect. The effect of the neuropeptide known as CCK is sensational. And anyone who wants to lose weight needs to understand it. As soon as the food you eat finishes being digested in the stomach, it is emptied into the beginning of the small intestine, known as the duodenum. That triggers the release of CCK, which suddenly pours into the bloodstream and acts on your vagus nerve to send the message to your brain cells.

"That message tells your brain that you aren't hungry anymore. As soon as the brain gets that news, you lose all interest in food. That's it! The meal is over. That's all you're going to eat until next time. It's like your appetite was hit over the head with a sledgehammer. As soon as the CCK takes hold, you fall back in your chair and you get that 'I-couldn't-eat-another-bite-if-my-life-depended-on-it' feeling. The 'Cholecystokinin Effect' in its most pronounced form is what most people experience after a nice big Thanksgiving dinner. It usually grabs them in the middle of the second piece of pumpkin pie. The CCK may save fat people from getting even fatter, but the only problem is that underweight people seem to be even more sensitive to it.''

Rick shrugged his shoulders. "Wow! That's amazing! I would never have imagined anything like that existed. But what can we do about it?''

"Well, we can't stop it. It's a built-in mechanism in our bodies. But we can try to work around it, at least to postpone it long enough so that we can get our quota of calories under our belt before it shuts off our ability to eat. But we have another enemy of weight gain to deal with at the same time—and we can fight it with the same weapons we use against CCK.''

That other built-in obstacle to gaining weight is a strange and exotic instinct that all human beings have—but very few people are even remotely aware of. It's known among scientists as the "Opioid Feeding Drive,'' or OFD.[3] (We medical doctors like to use abbreviations for these big words—it makes life a little easier.)

It works like this. Aside from the fact that you may get hungry as mealtime approaches, you also begin to feel a bit tense and restless. You may find it hard to concentrate on your work. You feel sort of edgy and impatient. Finally, when you sit down and as you begin to eat, you slowly and gradually feel a sense of calm and relaxation descending on you. You have just experienced the opioid feeding drive. That's because, in addition to a feeling of hunger, humans feel tension and agitation when they get hungry. It's like they have to stop what they're doing and move in the direction of food. That may have been a leftover from the way things were millions of years ago when we needed a prodding to get out and hunt for something to eat.

It might have been just that restlessness that pushed us out of the warm cave and into the cold damp forest hunting for rabbits or squirrels for dinner. Now, 10,000 years later, that same urge pushes us toward the dinner table or the luncheon appointment.

You may have felt it on occasion when you went to a restaurant when you were hungry and the service was slow. That urge you had to kill the waiter was as much a result of your Opioid Feeding Drive as anything else. If you recall, you were probably much more tense than hungry. But once the food arrived, and you started eating, you gradually lost all interest in doing harm to your snail-like waiter.

After careful analysis, researchers have proven that eating has almost the same effect as getting a little dose of opium. When we are hungry, we are driven to search for a way to calm our restlessness, as an addict is driven to search for opium. That's why it's called the Opioid Feeding Drive—"opioid" means "like opium." When we eat, we feel calmer and our compulsion to eat gradually disappears.

But that's a problem for us. If we are trying to gain weight, we want to keep that Opioid Feeding Drive going as long as possible. On the other hand, the folks who want to lose weight try to shut it off quickly. That's why they eat slowly, as they wait for the opioid effect to build up and the pressure and restlessness to dissipate.

In all the books on losing weight the advice is the same: "eat slowly and chew your food carefully." Although hardly anyone who writes books on weight reduction even knows about either the Opioid Feeding Drive or cholecystokinin, simply by observation over the years everyone has noticed that you eat less if you eat slowly and chew deliberately and carefully. Now for the first time we can tell our overweight friends why slow-paced eating cuts their consumption. It's simple. It allows the Opioid Feeding Drive and the Cholecystokinin Effect to put the brakes on their appetite before they can munch their way through too many calories.

Well, we don't want either of those mechanisms to get in the way of our eating. We don't want the Opioid Feeding Drive to dissipate that pressure and restlessness to eat. We want to keep it going as long and as intensely as possible. We don't want that cholecystokinin to pour into our bloodstream and zap our vagus nerve and our brain so that we can't down another bite.[4]

So what do we do? Well, we do the opposite. We want to eat fast—but not too fast. Our idea is not to gulp our food—but we don't want to dawdle over our meals either. When you sit down to eat, eat seriously. Take advantage of the momentum of your Opioid Feeding Drive before your brain gets the full message that you're getting something to eat. Like a football player trying to make a goal—you want to run ahead of the opposing team that is trying to tackle you—and your appetite.

The secret is to eat methodically and steadily. Insofar as possible, leave the conversation and the socializing for after your meal. It can make a very big difference. If you take a few bites of pizza, for example, and stop to join in the discussion of the movie you saw last night, the pizza will make its way relentlessly into your stomach. Then, if you eat a few more bites and then stop to talk about what you are going to do on the weekend, the pizza will move out of your stomach before you finalize your plans for Saturday night. The moment that pizza hits your duodenum, it triggers a rush of cholecystokinin into your bloodstream and your appetite falls flat on its face.[5]

In the same way, as you chew and swallow, chew and swallow, the clock is ticking against you. As each second goes by, that vital "drive to eat" of your Opioid Feeding Drive becomes less and less. When enough time goes by, you lose your momentum, the fork begins to get heavy in your hand, and you find yourself pecking away at your meal. I'm sure you know what I mean—it's happened dozens of times to all of us.

If you like, try this experiment. Take a meal you eat routinely—lunch at work or supper at home—it can be any meal you eat the same way at the same time regularly. A couple of times, eat the usual way—chatting, listening to the conversation, taking part in the social aspects of the meal. Then the next couple of times, eat seriously. Sit down, start eating, and eat your way right through, from start to finish. Don't talk, don't think about anything else, just eat as if it were your number-one assignment. (Interestingly enough, if you want to gain weight, it is your number-one assignment.) Keep track of what you eat both ways—eating socially or eating with a purpose. You may be pleasantly surprised to find you can eat much more easily and consume many more calories if you eat seriously and methodically. You will find real benefits if you can manage to run ahead of your personal Opioid Feeding Drive and that relentless cholecystokinin clock.[6]

How much time do you have before these two effects slam the brakes on your appetite?[7] It varies from person to person, of course. Everyone is a little different. It also depends on the circumstances—on what you are eating, how hungry you are, where you are eating, and whom you are eating with. But on the average you have about 13 minutes from the time you take the first bite of food or the first sip of liquid before these two roadblocks are thrown up in your path.

It all adds up to one thing: take your eating very seriously. Specifically, keep this in mind. It's not only what we eat but how we eat it. For those of us who want to gain weight, it makes sense to consume the maximum number of calories at each meal. Remember, our calories are being drained away at the rate of 90 per minute even if we are only sitting there looking out the window. Simply walking or doing light housework can double the drain on our calories. So just sit down to each meal with a calm mind and a spirit of dedication. Eat, chew, swallow, eat, chew, swallow, and get the food into your stomach before the alarm bells go off in your brain telling you that some hormone has decided you've had enough to eat. Eat your way through each meal deliberately and methodically, from start to finish—as if your life depended on it. And—in a real sense—it does.

There's something else to think about. When you are underweight and finally decide that you are going to do something about it, you have to make a couple of adjustments. The first and most important adjustment is the emotional one. You have to change your way of thinking, your outlook on life, and your image of yourself. From the first moment that you decide to gain weight, you have to become a fanatic about gaining just as other people are fanatics about losing weight. From now on, as far as you are concerned, every calorie counts. There's no such thing as an insignificant calorie. And remember that what we think of as 5 little calories is actually 5000 calories, in the scientific sense.

In reality there is a "Caloric Bill of Rights"—all calories are created equal. If you can pick up 5 calories here and 10 calories there, at the end of the day you will have added as many as 200 calories that otherwise would have slipped away from you. And those extra 200 calories that you snag will give you an extra pound in less than 18 days.

One excellent technique you can really use to your advantage is "Bonus Calories." It's almost like playing a game where you are always the winner. All you have to do is read every label on everything you buy and look for those extra calories where you least expected them. Do it every day and you will gradually develop an eagle eye for "hidden calories." Here's an example:

Canned fruit is especially good for weight gainers. It has a combination of sweet-and-tart flavors that makes it easy to eat without being overly filling. But don't walk into the supermarket and grab the first can of peaches you see. If you want a pleasant surprise, look for the "Bonus Calories."

There are actually 2 different kinds of canned peaches usually sold these days. One is called "clingstone" or "cling," because the peach stone clings to the inside of the peach as it is removed. It leaves a kind of ragged hole where the stone used to be. The other kind is called "freestone," because it comes loose easily as the peach is pitted. The hole in the peach is smooth and round.

An interesting bit of trivia useful only on game shows? No. It's "Bonus Calories" all the way. A cup of canned "clingstone" peaches will give you 190 calories. But choose the "freestone" peaches (same brand) and you get 216 calories in exactly the same amount of peaches. That's about 13 percent more of a push toward your goal—and the price is the same and the space they take in your stomach is identical. If you can add "Bonus Calories" like this to everything you eat, you can eat 3,500 calories to put on each pound but it will only feel like you're consuming 3,000 calories because your diet will have 13 percent more calories in exactly the same type and amount of food.

Here's another example. Take something as simple as a slice of bread. Our basic choice of bread is going to be plain old-fashioned white bread. It has plenty of calories, goes down easily, and doesn't fill us too fast. But unlike calories, all white bread is not created equal. If you check the labels you will see that what looks like the same slice of bread can give you either 88 or 58 calories. That's a whopping 35 percent difference in each slice! And remember, both kinds take exactly the same effort to chew and swallow and digest.*

Back in chapter 3, we analyzed the general examples of the I-Want-To-Lose-Weight Lunch, the I-Just-Want-Lunch Lunch, and the Quick Weight-Gain Program Lunch. Now let's get down to specifics and see how we can eat exactly the same amount of breakfast and gain three times as much weight!

Here are two breakfasts. One is the typical American breakfast. Most underweight people have eaten it thousands of times. The other one is the "Enhanced Breakfast" that you can start eating tomorrow morning. Let's see how they add up. Here's the usual version first:

## TRADITIONAL BREAKFAST

6 ounces orange juice (frozen)—72 calories
1 egg (hard boiled or boiled)—82 calories
1 cup of corn flakes with 4 ounces milk—160 calories
1 piece of toast with 1 tsp. butter (or margarine)—90 calories
1 cup of coffee black—2 calories

*Total:* 406 calories

---

* This comparison refers to bread with same-size slices. It does not include so-called thin-sliced bread that those who want to lose weight may prefer.

## Quick Weight-Gain Program Enhanced Breakfast

6 ounces bottled grape juice—122 calories

1 egg (fried)—108 calories

1 cup of Grape Nuts with 4 ounces of Half & Half—575 calories

1 English muffin with 2 tablespoons butter (or margarine)—345 calories

1 cup of coffee with 1 ounce of cream and sugar—100 calories

*Total:* 1,250 calories

So by the simple process of applying what we have learned, we have more than tripled the calories in our breakfast. But that's only part of it. We have tripled the calories without increasing the amount of food we have to eat. There isn't one more mouthful in the Enhanced Breakfast than in the Traditional Breakfast. There is nothing more to chew and nothing more to swallow. But there is 300 percent more calories!

The secret lies in picking each item carefully and adding "Bonus Calories" at every stage. Select foods for their fat and starch/sugar (carbohydrate) content. Add butter or margarine or oil wherever you can. If you're worried about butter and cholesterol, use polyunsaturated margarine or polyunsaturated oil but get those precious fat calories into your diet any way you can.

What about the cup of coffee? Remember we said that coffee and tea don't carry their weight in the Quick Weight-Gain Program? That's true but there are always exceptions. For a lot of people life is not worth living without a cup of coffee or tea—especially in the morning. Now we know a cup of coffee or a cup of tea weighs in at a mere 2 puny calories—ordinarily not even worth the trouble to drink it. But if you add an ounce of Half & Half and some sugar you bring it up to a respectable 100 calories. And what you are actually doing is using the tea or coffee as a "Calorie-Carrier." Look at it this way. It's hard to sit down to a nice plate of cream and sugar. Even though you can get 120 calories from 3 tablespoons of sugar and 60 calories from 3 tablespoons of cream for a grand total of 200 calories, there's a problem. Sweetened cream is not exactly a gourmet delicacy. But if you slip it into a cup of coffee or tea, then it becomes a nice relaxing break from the day's usual grind. We'll see more examples of tasty "Calorie-Carriers" in chapters 14 and 15.

Another question? Cream in your tea? Yes, of course. That's the way our British cousins have been drinking it for hundreds of years—and medically it makes sense. The cream offsets the powerful tannic acid in the tea which can cause discomfort in tea drinkers. It also mellows the brew—and most important for us, puts on the pounds. So drink your tea the British way and you'll help yourself to reach your goal. And if you don't put cream in the brew, at least use milk. When it comes to calories, every little bit helps. And every little bit of sacrifice will bring you closer to your goal.

While we're talking about sacrifices, it's worthwhile putting things into perspective. Our overweight friends really have to sacrifice. They often go to bed hungry, they can't eat all those wonderful goodies at parties and barbecues, and they are always worried and guilty about something they ate or wanted to eat. On the other hand, one of our problems is forcing ourselves to eat appetizing and tantalizing delicacies and change our diet in the tiniest of ways so we can gain the weight we want quickly and easily.

Now let's take a look at lunch and see how to apply the same concepts there.

Here is a typical lunch for people who work:

### TRADITIONAL AT-WORK LUNCH-BOX LUNCH

2 slices white bread—130 calories
2 ounces smoked luncheon-type ham (2 slices)—70 calories
1 tablespoon mayonnaise—100 calories
2 leaves lettuce—3 calories
1 apple—75 calories
1 piece of white cake (from mix)—180 calories
8 ounces cola drink—108 calories

*Total:* 666 calories

## QUICK WEIGHT-GAIN PROGRAM AT-WORK LUNCH-BOX LUNCH

2 slices rye bread—182 calories

4 slices bacon (thick-sliced)—240 calories

3 tablespoons mayonnaise—300 calories

2 leaves lettuce—3 calories

¼ tomato sliced—8 calories

4 ounces dates—376 calories

1 piece of cake (frozen devil's food from super-
    market)—293 calories

8 ounces lemon-lime canned fruit drink—128 calories

*Total:* 1,530 calories

This is just one more illustration of the weight-gaining power of the Quick Weight-Gain Program. We have been able to eat an amazing 230 percent more calories in approximately the same meal. And all we did was follow the "Bonus Calories" concept to the letter. Instead of smoked pork in the form of ham we substituted the same kind of meat—smoked pork in the form of bacon. The basic difference is that bacon has more of what we need to gain weight: fat. Instead of white bread, we used higher-calorie rye bread. The difference was 52 calories—about a 30 percent improvement. If you positively hate rye bread you can substitute white bread, but you will lose calories in the process.

You notice that we go lightly on the tomatoes and lettuce—why fill up on high-fiber low-calorie trimmings? We want the heavy stuff! An extra tablespoon of mayonnaise adds 100 welcome calories more. For fruit, dried dates give us a nice caloric boost. We remembered that dried fruits have a lot more calories per ounce and it paid off. We were careful about selecting the most caloric piece of cake—it helped us. And we even gained a few points with a lemon-lime canned fruit drink.

Now, what if you don't like this menu—bacon-lettuce-and-tomato sandwich on rye bread with dates for the fruit and frozen devil's food cake for dessert? There are two answers to that question. The first answer is this:

As we go along, and specifically in chapters 14 and 15, you will find many alternative high-calorie foods that you can use to prepare your own menus. You'll be sure to find a lot of your favorites there. The second answer is even more interesting. If you are really serious about gaining weight—and now you know a lot more reasons why you should be—you may have to eat something from time to time that isn't exactly at the top of your nutritional hit parade. That doesn't mean that you're going to have to munch on sautéed snails and barbecued octopus. But if from time to time you come across something that isn't exactly your favorite, try to eat it just the same. Remember, overweight people eat some awful stuff in their desperate struggle to lose weight. All you have to do is eat some really good stuff that you may not have had a lot of before to help you gain weight.

The dates in the previous lunch are a good example. You may not be a big fan of dates, but they contain important amounts of sugar and carbohydrate. They will go a long way to advance your cause. But if you just can't stand them, you can substitute peaches that come in at about 216 calories instead of 376 calories for the same four ounces. Peaches will help you gain, but dates will do it faster. If peaches don't agree with you, almost any dried fruit will do. Remember, dried fruit is caloric dynamite. For example, a half cup of Thompson grapes will give you a measly 54 calories. But if those identical grapes are dried and become Thompson raisins, the same half cup will provide you with an amazing 212 calories. Just by getting rid of the water you have increased the caloric value 400 percent. As usual, it won't take you any more effort to eat the same amount of grapes after the water has been removed. And the big advantage is that you'll be getting 4 times the calories.

How about supper? You've seen all those articles and advertisements that insist that breakfast is the most important meal of the day? Well, they're wrong—at least for those of us who want to put on weight. Think of it this way. There is an old proverb for people who want to lose weight that says, "Eat breakfast like a king, eat lunch like a squire, and eat supper like a pauper." It's good advice if you want to lose weight. For some reason that no one understands, if we eat a lot before going to bed, it tends to put on weight. Maybe it's because our metabolism drops off while we're asleep or maybe it has to do with the fact that important glandular secretions like the thyroid and adrenals vary throughout the day and night. But the explanation isn't vital for us. What does matter is that one bite at night is worth two in the morning. So we should work hard to get as many calories as we possibly can from 5:00 P.M. to bedtime.

Let's start by taking a look at a Traditional Supper, the kind most people eat.

### TRADITIONAL SUPPER

> 8-ounce bowl of soup (onion soup from a prepared
>     mix)—34 calories
> T-bone steak trimmed of visible fat around edges, ¼
>     pound—254 calories
> Salad: iceberg lettuce 4 leaves with 2 tablespoons
>     French dressing—124 calories
> 1 baked potato (⅓ pound average)—90 calories
> ½ cup cut green beans (frozen)—21 calories
> 1 dinner roll—61 calories
> ½ cup chocolate pudding (dairy case)—150 calories

> *Total:* 734 calories

Remember this "typical supper" is not a weight-reduction diet. It includes steak, salad, soup, potato, a roll, two vegetables, and chocolate pudding for dessert. And all the items are "off the shelf"—they aren't "lo-cal" or dietetic. So it adds up to a typical 734 calories.

## QUICK WEIGHT-GAIN PROGRAM SUPPER

8-ounce bowl of soup (ready-to-serve canned split pea
    soup with ham)—186 calories

T-bone steak, untrimmed, ¼ pound with 1 tablespoon
    melted butter (or margarine) on steak—639 calories

Salad: ½ California avocado with 2 tablespoons bottled
    Italian dressing—350 calories

1 cup mashed potatoes, with milk and butter (or marga-
    rine) added—200 calories

½ cup green peas in butter sauce (frozen)—90 calories

½ cup cut green beans in mushroom sauce (frozen)—
    100 calories

1 crescent roll with 1 tablespoon butter (or margarine)—
    202 calories

Apple pie, 4-ounce slice—415 calories

*Total:* 2,182 calories

This is another example of "Bonus Calories." It takes approximately the same number of bites to eat these two meals. They are
almost identical except that the Quick Weight-Gain Program Supper
has every item carefully chosen for its "Bonus Calories," primarily
in the form of fat. So by eating almost the same meal, we are getting
300 percent more calories for our efforts.

And I know what you are going to ask: Why do I specify a
California avocado? Am I partial just because I'm a Californian?
No. It's just that a California avocado gives you 86 more calories
in each avocado—on the average. Why? Because of the higher oil
content. Avocados from California are a different variety from
their Florida cousins and give you more calories in each bite. This
is a perfect way to use "Bonus Calories." You're eating exactly
the same amount of the identical food and yet you're getting at
least 25 percent more calories. That's really painless progress. Onward and upward!

The Quick Weight-Gain Program way is the best way ever devised for gaining weight. It is simple, sure, and trouble-free. But occasionally we encounter the tiniest pebbles in our path as we work to put on the pounds. Jennifer tells about one example:

She was a striking redhead—striking in two ways. Her bright red, nearly crimson, hair made her bright green eyes seem almost iridescent. She was tall and stately, but at 5 feet 7 inches her 106 pounds made her stand out in a way that she never intended. With a body mass index of 16.67 she was much too thin. And this is what she was worried about:

"You know, Doctor, I feel like a little ashamed now that I've decided to put on weight. You know, I'm an Account Executive in a big advertising agency and there are a lot of people constantly coming and going."

"What kind of people, Jennifer?"

"Well, there are clients and then the people I work with and the graphic artists on contract and the TV people. Some days I must talk to 75 people—at least. And I feel funny about it. I mean, if I gain weight—and I really need to gain—it's going to be embarrassing. All these dozens of people are going to see me change right before their eyes and I don't know how to explain it or anything. I'm afraid they're going to make fun of me and crack a lot of dumb jokes and all that. What should I do?"

"You should do exactly what makes you feel the most comfortable, of course. But most of my patients have decided to tell everyone they know that they are trying to make a sincere effort to gain weight. I don't know anyone who has ever regretted it."

Jennifer brightened up.

"I'll try it, Doctor! After all, overweight people announce to the world that they are on a diet and they repeat it everywhere they go! There should be equal rights for us skinny folks!"

"You've got the right idea! And you just may discover a very interesting secret in the process. Let me know how it works out."

A week later, at her next visit, Jennifer was all smiles.

"How did it work?"

"Like magic, Doctor. Like pure magic! I told absolutely everyone—even the guys in the mailroom! And now I know why you encouraged me to tell the world about my new project."

It was my turn to smile. "So you discovered the secret?"

"I sure did! Not too many people really know how to lose weight but everyone and his brother is an expert on gaining weight! And they really want to help. I told my supervisor about it and he must have told the president of the agency, Mr. Cooper. Mr. Cooper never comes out of his office but that same afternoon he came out, came into my office and congratulated me. Then he told me what his grandmother did to help him and his brother to gain weight when they were little. It was a cod liver oil and vitamin $B_1$ mixture that the druggist in their little town made up. He even wrote it down for me. I couldn't believe it! Of course, I'm sure that vitamins can't do people any good."

"Don't be so sure, Jennifer. We'll talk about that later on.* But you found out what I was talking about?"

"I certainly did, Doctor. Everyone was so supportive and so helpful. And everyone had a useful suggestion. You know, if you're trying to lose weight sometimes people get impatient with you because they're trying to lose weight too and they're kind of tense about it. But gain weight? That's different! At least half the people I told had exactly the same reaction."

"What was that?"

"They said: 'Wow! I only wish I had that problem myself!' But

* We'll check into this and other vitamin combinations that may help us in chapter 9.

I'm really glad I did it. Everyone is so nice and they keep encouraging me every time I see them.''

And that's the way it happens. Unless you have some very special reason to keep your weight-gaining project a secret, tell your friends and family and coworkers about it. You'll be pleasantly surprised and delighted with their response. You can usually depend on them to come up with interesting suggestions and hints about methods that have helped other people. And when you get invitations to dinner or to parties or to picnics, you won't have to put up with the usual low-calorie, low-fat, low-carbohydrate menus that are so fashionable these days—and so useless in our weight-gaining program. That's something else that helped Jennifer:

"The thing I didn't expect was the one thing that probably helped me the most, Doctor."

"What was that?"

"What I like to call the 'emergency rations.' You know how hard it is to get the kind of food we need on this diet. Well, so many people started bringing me special foods. Like our Puerto Rican messenger boy brought me some fried bananas that his mother had made up. And one of the other account executives was on a business trip to San Francisco and she brought me some special high calorie crackers from a hippie health food store there. And now when I get invited to a party they always have what they call 'Jennifer's Table.' Sometimes it's a separate little folding table with my kind of food. You know, fried food and plenty of starches and sugars and the kinds of things they know I need. And they have special desserts for me—cheesecake made with real creamy cheese and that sort of thing.

"And when I go out on a date, sometimes it's really amusing. It's like the different men I go out with are sort of competing to see who can take me to the most fattening restaurant. Last Friday a fellow I've known for years, Gene, took me to a place called 'Fat Freddie's Barbecue and Pizza Palace.' Freddie, the owner, must have weighed 300 pounds and Gene called him over to our table.

"He said, 'I'll have a small whole-wheat pizza with low-fat mozzarella cheese and tomatoes.' Then Freddie said, 'The same for the lady?' Then Gene laughed and said, 'No sir! Bring her just exactly what you eat for dinner every night!'

"Freddie got very serious and disappeared into the kitchen. In about ten minutes he came out with Gene's small pizza and a teenie-weenie salad for me. Gene's eyes almost popped out of his head. Then he realized what had happened and he started laughing.

" 'My mistake, Freddie. Let's start all over again. Don't bring her what you're eating now. Bring her what you used to eat before you went on a diet.'

"Freddie nodded and disappeared back into the kitchen. When he finally came out, he was carrying a pizza that looked like a tabletop and was at least three inches thick. He laid it down on the table with a thud and I could see him drool as he looked at it. I couldn't eat it all, of course, but I'm sure what I managed to eat did me a lot of good."

So don't be afraid to tell everyone about your new weight-gaining plan. You have everything in the world to gain—and nothing whatsoever to lose.

**Chapter Seven**

# Putting The Program to Work for You: More Calories with Every Bite

**N**ow that we understand how our bodies operate to keep us underweight, we can begin to take definite steps to put on weight once and for all—and to keep it on. Let's get right down to business with the Quick Weight-Gain Program.

As always, the fundamental idea is to utilize foods that have the greatest number of calories in the smallest possible space. As we have seen, the food type that does that best is fat. Before we go any further, please get rid of any fear of fat that may linger in your mind. Without going into all the details of the "cholesterol controversy," consider only these important facts:

1. The American diet, from 1776 to 1949, was loaded with saturated animal fat. We used lard as the principal shortening, we ate immense amounts of fatty meat, including pork and sausages of all kinds. We consumed eggs by the trillions and drank milk and ate ice cream by the billions of tons. In spite of all of this, the first significant cases of heart attacks were reported in the United States in 1912—136 years after the massive consumption of fat and cholesterol began.[1]

2. Since 1949 we have been on an antifat campaign never before seen in the history of the world.[2] No eggs! No milk! No cream! No meat! No animal fat! Fat consumption

dropped 30 percent. And as a result we have eliminated heart attacks? What a joke! Between 1949 and 1973, the number of deaths from heart attacks doubled![3] Today and every day, almost 3,000 Americans will clutch their chests, suddenly collapse, and die an excruciating death from a heart attack. As you read this page, at least two innocent victims will succumb as their heart muscle sputters and dies. Tragically, the incidence of heart attacks has shown no significant decrease in spite of the hysterical antifat campaign.

**3.** Other countries in the world—France, Italy, and Spain to name only three—have diets much higher in fat than we do—and a much lower incidence of heart attacks.

**4.** You will only be on a relatively high-fat diet for six months or so. Even the most fanatic enemy of fat agrees that it takes years and years—decades—of eating massive amounts of fat to produce even the slightest hazard to your health.

**5.** The risk of death and serious disease as a direct result of being underweight is far greater than that of even a lifetime of a high-fat diet.

**6.** If you are concerned about cholesterol, restrict your fat intake to unsaturated fats like corn oil, safflower oil, olive oil, etc.

**7.** What about cholesterol? As far as cholesterol is concerned, everyone is agreed that there are at least two forms of cholesterol. (It wasn't so long ago that we thought there was only one.) There is ''high-density cholesterol'' and ''low-density cholesterol.'' One is supposed to be ''good'' for you and the other is supposed to be ''bad'' for you. As you can see we still have a lot to learn about cholesterol. But the cholesterol story goes even deeper than that. If all the cholesterol were suddenly and magically drained from your body, you would die in that instant. Why? Because such vital organs as your eyes, brain, liver, testicles, and ovaries are replete with cholesterol. If you don't consume enough cholesterol, your body will manufacture it synthetically.

So have no fear. Your most important goal from the point of view of your health—and your very survival—is to gain weight. The fat that you are going to eat is the only way to accomplish that goal. You owe it to yourself and your family to do everything you possibly can to attain a normal weight as soon as possible.

Now that we have that out of the way, let's get down to business. What's for breakfast? Maybe nothing. And maybe something. We've all heard that breakfast is the "most important meal of the day"— and well it may be to some people. But if we want to gain weight, it can be a mixed blessing. If you eat a big breakfast in the belief that it will help you gain weight it may actually cut down on your total caloric consumption for the day. How? Like this:

A lot of people don't really have a big appetite for break-fast—or the time to eat what they should or as much as they should. For those of us who work, it's up and out of bed, wash and dress, and then eat something with one eye on the clock. There isn't usually time to select the food carefully or to eat it the way we should. What's the answer? Well, a popular meal in England is called "The Ploughman's Lunch." In this case we have "The Working-Person's Breakfast." The idea is to offer a good, appe-tizing, high-calorie meal that you can prepare easily and eat with-out dawdling. That's the perfect way you get your calories on time *and* you get to work on time.

Breakfast often starts with orange juice. But let's enhance it by adding a tablespoon of sugar for an extra 40 calories. Then it's on to the main course.

One of the best friends of the "The Working-Person's Break-fast" is the toaster-pastry. These are nice little fruit- or chocolate-filled pastries that you can just pop in your toaster as you buzz around the kitchen in the morning.

The next item is a beverage. Regular tea or coffee won't help you calorie-wise but a lot of folks depend on the caffeine in their morning coffee or tea to get them going to face the new day. The problem is that we'd be better off getting calories from everything, including our morning drink. Although most people don't realize it, you can get almost the same jump-start from chocolate drinks as you can from coffee. A good strong cup of coffee or tea contains about 90 milligrams of caffeine or the equivalent. A cup of cocoa made from 1 ounce of powdered cocoa contains about 50 milligrams of caffeine. So a cup or two of cocoa or chocolate milk should get you raring to go in the morning—and add pounds at the same time. What if you don't care for cocoa? No problem. A good choice is one of those ready-made coffee drinks from the dairy case. They give you coffee taste, caffeine push, and extra calories all in the same swallow. You can finish off with a slice of bread. An English muffin gives you the most calories per bite—if you like it. Add a couple of tablespoons of butter or margarine and a couple of tablespoons of jam or jelly and you have a 495-calorie package.

## THE QUICK WEIGHT-GAIN PROGRAM
## WORKING-PERSON'S BREAKFAST

> 1 typical "toaster-pastry" (Pop-Tart or similar)—205 calories
> 1 English muffin—145 calories, *with*
> 2 tablespoons of margarine (unsaturated)—200 calories, *and*
> 2 tablespoons of jelly or jam—150 calories
>
> *Total:* 1,110 to 1,140 calories (depending on your choice of cocoa or prepared coffee mix)

Remember, this is the basic framework of a "got-to-go-to-work" breakfast. You can substitute various other food items for the ones in the example. It's just a matter of plugging in your favorite foods from a long list of possibilities. That's how you will construct custom-made meals that fit your tastes perfectly—and put on the pounds like never before.

Now, if you don't have to rush off to work every morning—or for those nice Saturday and Sunday morning breakfasts for working folks—here is the outline for the Quick Weight-Gain Program Stay-At-Home Breakfast. That gives you the opportunity to add even more calories and gain weight even faster. Here's an example:

You can start out with the same "enhanced" orange juice and cocoa or coffee mix. But since you don't have to rush off to work, you can fry yourself a few slices of bacon. First of all, remember, there are two kinds of meat called bacon. One is good old American bacon, which is the kind we want to eat. It is about 70 percent fat and "good fat" in the sense that it goes down easily and tastes great. Remember, that's our challenge. Eating 100 percent fat works against us by killing our appetite on the spot. Even 80 percent fat is hard to take. But 70 percent in a tasty and palatable form will go a long way toward helping us achieve our goal.

But beware! There is another kind of bacon called "Canadian bacon." That's fine for folks who want to lose weight. It's barely 14 percent fat and it won't do us any good at all. There's something else to look out for when you're shopping for bacon. There is a tremendous variation in the caloric content between brands. The slice of bacon that looks almost the same can have as few as 100 calories or as many as 225 calories. Let's assume that our slice has about 175 calories in each slice although if you look carefully you may do even better.

## THE QUICK WEIGHT-GAIN PROGRAM STAY-AT-HOME BREAKFAST

1 8-ounce glass of fresh orange juice with 1 teaspoon
    sugar—150 calories

1 8-ounce cup of cocoa from a mix (hot or cold)—260
    calories

    or

1 8-ounce cup of prepared coffee mix ("Instant Break-
    fast" type of drink)—290 calories

4 slices of bacon—700 calories

2 eggs fried—215 calories

1 English muffin—145 calories, with

2 tablespoons of margarine (unsaturated)—200 calories,
   *and*
2 tablespoons of jelly or jam—150 calories

*Total:* 1,820 or 1,850 calories (depending on your
   choice of cocoa or prepared coffee mix)

If you substitute pork sausage for the bacon, you'll only cut the calories by 340 or so, and you can add a little variety to your menus.

As you can see, there is plenty of room for ingenuity and inventiveness in this project. If you come across any tricks or hints that have been particularly useful to you, I'd be delighted to hear about them. Just drop me a line at this address: Dr. David Reuben, M.D., c/o Harold Matson Co., 276 Fifth Avenue, New York, N.Y. 10001. The hints that helped you might well help someone else to gain the weight they need so much.

In the last chapter we saw the framework for the Quick Weight-Gain Program At-Work Lunch-Box Lunch. But not everyone takes their lunch to work. Some people who don't go to work eat lunch at home. A lot of people who work eat at restaurants or order food to take out or be delivered. And nowadays there are more and more working people who work at home. Folks in these groups have special opportunities and sometimes special problems. For those people we have the basic Quick Weight-Gain Program Stay-At-Home Lunch. It's a wonderful opportunity to really advance our cause.

One of the nice things about eating lunch at home is that we have complete control of the situation and we can structure everything carefully so that it works in our favor. In a certain sense, one lunch at home is worth two lunches at work. And here's another clue. Don't engage in any strenuous exercise for at least an hour before lunch. We want our liver to be full of glycogen so that when we eat, all our calories will be sent directly to be stored as extra weight, not held temporarily in the liver to be used for physical activity.

Let's get started. If you like soup, this is an opportunity for you. Soup, like many liquids including tea and coffee, is an excellent vehicle for calories. You can load up a nice bowl of soup with dozens and dozens of extra calories and they just slide right down your throat. You'll hardly even notice them—until they give you that pleasant surprise when you step on the scale.

Even if you don't particularly care for soup it's worth trying to find one that you can go with—just for the very real caloric benefits it offers. And don't worry about eating hot soup during warm weather. Take advantage of this little-known fact: when the weather is hot, a hot beverage will actually cool you off!

Another advantage of soup—especially if you eat it at home—is that it's easy to enhance. That is, if you choose cream soup. Most canned cream soups can take a tablespoon or two of butter, margarine, or olive oil and end up tasting even better than when they came out of the can. By the way, we say "out of the can" based on the assumption that few people these days take the time and trouble to make their own soup. So start off with soup and be sure to add a tablespoon of butter, margarine, or oil according to your preference. You'll get your meal off to a turbocharged start.

Salad is the next course and that's another benefit of eating at home. You can take your salad in a lunch box or order it in a restaurant, but it just isn't the same. At home you can put together a "custom-made" salad—enhanced to the limit—and get the maximum advantage from it.

## The Quick Weight-Gain Program Stay-At-Home Lunch

8-ounce bowl of soup (ready-to-serve canned cream of mushroom) with 1 tablespoon of butter, margarine, or oil—317 calories

Waldorf Salad: 2 apples peeled and cut in eighths, 4 tablespoons mayonnaise, and ½ cup walnuts—925 calories

2 pork chops—520 calories

Fried potatoes—French fried or hash brown, 3½-ounce serving—270 calories

Coconut Creme Pie, 4-ounce slice—480 calories

*Total:* 2,512 calories

But remember one very important principle: If you can't eat everything in a typical menu, just pick out the highest-calorie foods and eat them. That way you'll get the most benefit with the least work.

Of course this is only a sample Quick Weight-Gain Program Stay-At-Home Lunch menu. You'll find more just right for you in chapter 14. But how about those of us who can't stay home and can't or don't want to bring a lunch box? How do we manage to eat in restaurants or company cafeterias and still gain weight? To be honest, it's a challenge, more in company dining rooms than in restaurants. But the Quick Weight-Gain Program meets all challenges, and eating in the company dining room, college cafeteria, or military base is no problem for us. Let's take an example—the typical company dining room or college cafeteria.

The basic principle here—as we know by now—is to add as much low-volume, high-calorie components to your diet. In most cases that means "fat." But where do we find fat in a cafeteria? Fortunately it is all around us—if we can just look for it. Let's check out the kind of lunch you might find in just such a mass-feeding place and see how we can turn it to our advantage. Here's the standard-type meal the way it's served; later we'll see how we can enhance it on the spot.

## TYPICAL COMPANY OR COLLEGE CAFETERIA LUNCH

Beef vegetable soup, 8 ounces—75 calories
Spaghetti with tomato sauce, ½ cup—150 calories
Mixed salad with 2 tablespoons French dressing—130
    calories
Zucchini boiled, ½ cup—15 calories
Peas, ½ cup—60 calories
White bread, 1 slice—75 calories
Butter, ½ tablespoon—50 calories
Gelatin Dessert, ½ cup—80 calories

*Total:* 635 calories

Do you wonder how anyone survives on that kind of lunch? Good question. And the next question is what can we do about it? The answer is: plenty. Let's get started!

Our basic resources are right there in the cafeteria line. All we have to do is take a clue from a famous performance by the actor Jimmy Stewart. The scene was New York City during the terrible economic depression of the 1930s. Jimmy was all alone in New York, down on his luck, and with almost no money. Worst of all, he was hungry. So he strolled into an unusual type of restaurant known as the Automat. Along one wall, there were dozens of little boxes with glass doors like post office boxes. Each one had a slot to insert a coin and behind each door was a sandwich or a salad or a piece of pie. All the customer had to do was insert a quarter or a dime, open the door, and take out the food item he wanted. Jimmy had no money, but he was a thinker. He took a coffee mug—no charge. Then he filled it half with hot water—no charge. Then he added ketchup, mustard, and any other seasoning that was available and free. He then sat down like any other customer, stirred it leisurely with a spoon and drank it calmly. He got his calories—no charge.

Well, that's not exactly our problem. We're willing to pay, but we have to use our ingenuity to make mass food into weight-gaining food. Taking our cue from Jimmy Stewart, here we go!

In most cafeteria settings, both butter or margarine and salad oil are available—either free or at a small extra charge. Take advantage of them—they are the concentrated calories we need. Remember we are burning 1.5 calories a minute just sitting around. If we are going to really gain weight, we have to get as many calories as we can with each meal. We can't afford a single wishy-washy low-calorie meal. We have to replenish our stores of energy at every opportunity.

If we were ordering in a restaurant or cooking for ourselves, we'd choose a "cream" soup—cream of mushroom, cream of chicken, etc. But at an in-house restaurant we can't always pick and choose. So let's stay with beef vegetable soup, which proves that we can add calories to anything except a concrete block, if we have to.

## THE QUICK WEIGHT-GAIN PROGRAM ENHANCED COMPANY OR COLLEGE CAFETERIA LUNCH

Beef vegetable soup, 8 ounces—75 calories. Add 2 tablespoons of butter or salad oil to bring it up to 275 calories.

Spaghetti with tomato sauce, ½ cup—150 calories. Add plenty of grated cheese. If you can add 2 ounces of cheese you will raise the energy value to 390 calories.

Mixed salad with 2 tablespoons French dressing—130 calories. Add at least one ounce of grated cheese and you will bring it up to 250 calories. Then crumble an ounce of potato chips (available from vending machines almost everywhere) over the salad for another 160 calories. Now your salad is worth a more respectable 410 calories.

Zucchini, boiled, ½ cup—15 calories. Your best bet is to add 2 tablespoons of butter or margarine or salad oil to bring it up to 215 calories.

Peas, ½ cup—60 calories. Your best bet is—the same. Add 2 tablespoons of butter or margarine or salad oil to bring it up to 260 calories.

White bread, 1 slice—75 calories. Spread 2 tablespoons of jelly or jam on that slice of bread to bring it up to 175 calories.

Butter, ½ tablespoon—50 calories. Double the butter to 1 tablespoon—that makes it 100 calories.

Gelatin Dessert, ½ cup—80 calories. Don't pick a gelatin dessert. Almost every mass-feeding restaurant has a high-calorie dessert available. Try a nice piece of chocolate cake instead at 180 calories. If you can, add a scoop of ice cream at 130 calories or so. If

you can't order ice cream, then look for an ice
cream bar at a vending machine for about the same
number of calories. Total for dessert: 310 calories.

*Total:* 2,135 calories

Incidentally, that's another weapon we can use to defend ourselves from the slim offerings at company or college cafeterias. We
can always turn to vending machines for ''emergency rations'' to
supplement undercaloried meals. (For more hints on ''emergency
rations,'' check chapter 9.)

The Typical Company or College Cafeteria Lunch was going
to leave us with a puny 635 calories—calories that would be totally dissipated in a mere 7 hours if we just sat still. By following
the example of Jimmy Stewart, we have converted it into something that we can be proud of—a meal that will add ounces and
pounds to our body weight and bring us that much closer to our
goal.

We've made pretty good progress in dealing with the problems
of those of us who have to bring our lunch to work, those who can
enjoy the luxury of eating at home, and those who have to eat in
company or college cafeterias. There's just one more major group
that we have to work for—the millions of people who eat lunch at a
restaurant every working day. Those folks have special challenges.
First they have to think of the cost of their lunch. Eating out every
day isn't cheap and the temptation—understandably—is to buy the
most economical lunch that will fill you until dinnertime. The next
constraint is time. If you have an hour for lunch, that doesn't mean
an hour to eat. By the time you get to the crowded restaurant,
manage to attract the attention of a waiter or waitress, order your
lunch, get served, and begin eating, you may only have minutes
before you have to be on your way back to the job. And the third
problem is quality. It may be hard to find a clean restaurant with
reasonable prices and good-quality food close enough to where you
work. But if you do decide to eat your lunch in a restaurant, here's
about what you can expect:

## TYPICAL LUNCH-HOUR RESTAURANT LUNCH

1 hamburger, 3 ounces on bun with lettuce, ketchup, and
   pickles—365 calories
French-fried potatoes, 10 pieces—150 calories
1 cola drink, 8 ounces—100 calories
Ice cream, ½ cup—130 calories

*Total:* 745 calories

That will keep your body functioning for a bare 8 hours. At the first minute of the ninth hour you will start burning up your fat reserves and begin to lose weight!

Unfortunately the hamburger-fries-soft-drink routine doesn't give us too much to work with as far as enhancement goes. If we want to do better than that, our choices are few. We can bring our lunch, eat in the company cafeteria (if there is one), or improvise the best we can in a commercial restaurant. Three tough choices. But there is a fourth choice that some of us can take advantage of. If we work in a place with an understanding and cooperative employer or if we have our own store or shop, we can have all the advantages of eating at home and none of the disadvantages of bringing our lunch. All we need is a small microwave oven and a small refrigerator with a tiny freezer. (If there is a supermarket very close by, we don't even need the freezer.)

All we have to do is stock a few carefully selected frozen dinners and other selected frozen goodies and heat them in the microwave at the appropriate time. Working together we can even figure out how to get the full-calorie weight-gaining meal that we need—all from the microwave and the freezer.

Let's take a look at a typical "Microwave-Puts-on-the-Pounds" Lunch.

## THE QUICK WEIGHT-GAIN PROGRAM
## MICROWAVE-PUTS-ON-THE-POUNDS LUNCH

Frozen Mexican dinner—570 calories

Sour cream, 8 tablespoons (to be spread over tacos, en-
chiladas, etc., as in typical Mexican dinner)—240
calories

Frozen apple turnover—290 calories

Chocolate milk drink, 8 ounces, from dairy case—290
calories

*Total:* 1,390 calories

That's almost twice as many calories as you get in the Typical
Lunch-Hour Restaurant Lunch—and probably a lot more appetizing. And microwaving your lunch has a very special appeal. The
food is fresh and hot and attractive. The selection is vast, and if
you stock several varieties of meals you'll always find just the one
that fits your mood. That's an important point. You will always eat
the most if you are eating something you really like. When it
comes to frozen dinners, you can select from Chinese, Italian, German, fish, shrimp, turkey, Mexican, and almost anything else. So
if one day you just have a taste for chicken chow mein—and you
feel you can eat a double serving—you won't have to settle for
whatever the local restaurant is featuring that day. Just step to the
freezer, snap on the microwave, pop in your meal, and you'll enjoy
just what you wanted.

But what if you can't have the use of those two wonderful
appliances? Don't worry, we can work out a solution to almost every
problem. These days the world is full of take-out and "we-bring-it-
to-you" restaurants. You can order almost anything, have it delivered, and enhance it on the spot. Some of the handiest tools to raise
the calories of "express" meals—the ones that roll up to your office
or factory door—can be kept in the back of a desk drawer or toolbox.
Here are some examples:

1. Mayonnaise. Collect those little foil packets of mayonnaise that they give at fast food places or sell at your supermarket. They keep without refrigeration (until you open them) and remember each tablespoon will add 100 calories to your diet. You can add the mayonnaise to French fries, submarine, torpedo, or ''Poor Boy'' sandwiches, hamburgers, fried chicken, or anything else you can think of.

2. Imitation bacon bits. A tablespoon adds 40 extra calories and they are so light you hardly notice them. But every calorie counts. Add those bits of flavor to salads, pizza, sandwiches, hamburgers, and all the rest.

3. Vienna sausage. Those nice little sausages that come in handy cans with the lift-off top can reinforce the calories of take-out foods like nothing else. Each little sausage is worth about 45 calories. Add them to pizza, salads, sandwiches, and anything else you can think of. They will add calories with hardly any trouble.

4. Cheese spreads. Many of these do not have to be refrigerated and have as many as 80 calories per ounce. There are even some that come in an aerosol can so you can squirt them onto whatever seems appropriate.

5. Deviled ham. That nice little can of deviled ham will give you about 95 calories for each ounce you add to your take-out meal.

That's the key. Put your ingenuity to work, and you'll find plenty of places to slip in these and other calorie boosters and watch the calories add up. Once you are turned on to the concept of seriously gaining weight, you will be amazed and delighted at how fast the ideas will spring into your mind. You will come up with new and exciting ways to augment every meal and reach your goal faster than ever.

But what if you can't have a freezer and a microwave? What if there is no company cafeteria? What if you can't go home for lunch?

What if your only alternative is to pick the best restaurant you can find and do the best you can there? Well, let's go out to lunch again and see how we can enhance the calorie content.

Let's try Mexican food again although the same basic principles will work fine with almost any full-fledged cuisine like Italian, German, French, Chinese, etc. But Mexican food is easy to work with. It is intrinsically high in fat and also has enough ''body'' to it that we can add our own calories. And remember, the basic ingredients for calorie enhancement are usually right there on your table. Almost invariably you will find sugar freely available, along with butter or margarine. You can always ask for a little bottle of oil for your salad. Interestingly enough, most restaurants don't charge extra for extra oil, although that is one of the most expensive ingredients in the kitchen. Here's a typical Mexican restaurant lunch—before we start to augment it.

## THE TYPICAL MEXICAN
## LUNCH-HOUR RESTAURANT LUNCH

1 cup chile con carne with beans—300 calories
2 beef tamales—160 calories
1 8-ounce glass root beer, lemon-lime, or grapefruit soft
    drink—110 calories
Mexican custard dessert ''flan,'' ½ cup—140 calories

*Total:* 710 calories

Now here's our enhanced version:

## THE QUICK WEIGHT-GAIN PROGRAM ENHANCED
## MEXICAN LUNCH-HOUR RESTAURANT LUNCH

1 cup chile con carne without beans. Add 2 tablespoons
    of salad oil, butter, or margarine to the chile con carne
    after it is served to you at your table—780 calories
½ cup refried beans. Add 1 tablespoon of salad oil, but-
    ter, or margarine after it is served to you at your
    table—240 calories

2 beef tamales with sauce—280 calories

1 8-ounce glass root beer, lemon-lime, or grapefruit soft
    drink. Add 1 tablespoon of sugar to drink—brown
    sugar for the root beer and regular sugar for the cit-
    rus drinks—150 calories

1 piece of cake (1/12 of the cake), chocolate, coconut,
    yellow, or cheesecake—225 calories

1 scoop of ice cream—140 calories

*Total:* 1,815 calories

Let's see how we added calories simply and easily—and without increasing the price of the meal.

Starting with the chile con carne, we can add extra fat since the other ingredients will soak it up so that it disappears almost completely. We get more calories—and more food—if we order the refried beans separately. Refried beans will also easily absorb an extra tablespoon of salad oil, butter, or margarine. (By the way they don't call them "refried" beans because they are fried twice. The Spanish word *refrito* merely means "thoroughly fried." That may come in handy in the next trivia contest.) Depending on your taste, you may even want to add more fat for more calories. You don't have to add very much to the beef tamales—they can stand pretty well on their own.

And here's something interesting for root beer fans. A lot of the commercial root beer sold just doesn't have the same old-time flavor of the original home-brewed variety. But you can bring back most of the real authentic flavor just by adding a teaspoon of brown sugar to each glass. Stir well and you will really be in for a taste treat—and the extra caloric bonus. The citrus-flavored drinks tend to be a little on the tart side and they can absorb a spoonful of sugar without suffering very much. Those extra calories are welcome too.

So we managed about 250 percent more calories than the Typical Lunch-Hour Restaurant Lunch and almost 25 percent more calories than the Quick Weight-Gain Program Microwave-Puts-on-the-Pounds Lunch. Of course, the actual calories will vary from day to day depending on the exact food items we include. But you can be sure of one thing—each and every Quick Weight-Gain Program Enhanced Lunch-Hour Restaurant Lunch and each and every Quick Weight-Gain Program Microwave-Puts-on-the-Pounds Lunch will leave the standard everyday diets choking in the dust.

You can apply exactly the same concepts to having dinner at a restaurant. And keep in mind that it doesn't have to be a fancy silver-spoon place. At most of the fast-food restaurants you can enhance the menus on the spot enough to advance your cause. If you're eating pizza ask for double (or triple) cheese—and just watch closely to make sure that you're getting everything you ask for—and pay for. At fried chicken restaurants make sure you get plain old fried chicken. Many places fry their chicken in "pressure fryers." These are brilliant inventions that are a cross between a fryer and a pressure cooker. Many of them tend to cut down on the amount of oil that the breading on the chicken absorbs. That's good news for overweight people—it helps them lose weight. But we want all the calories we can get and the more shortening that sticks to the chicken, the more weight that will stick to our ribs. (Speaking of ribs, if you like spareribs, you're in luck. A mere 4 ounces of spareribs will give you an impressive 400 calories. Add ¼ cup of barbecue sauce and you're looking at 500 delicious calories.)

If we are going to gain weight away from home, there are two things that will help us tremendously. First, always keep in mind the idea that what we eat has to be appetizing. No matter how many calories an item contains, if it's not taste tempting, we won't want to eat enough of it to make a real difference. Secondly, we have to constantly use our ingenuity to find ways to enhance restaurant food, take-out food, or supermarket food to build in more and more calories.

To make things easier you can check with the distinguished members of the Quick Weight-Gain Program 400 Society. These are a handy list of foods that you are likely to find on restaurant menus. They qualify for membership in the club because a 4-ounce serving of each one will give you about 400 calories. (Keep in mind that all caloric values are approximate, since the moisture content, preparation, and many other factors can affect the exact measurement.) When you give your order to the waiter, try to include at least one of these if you can.

1. Lamb chops
2. Sweetbreads (beef)
3. Hot dogs
4. Polish sausage
5. Pork roast
6. Fried chicken
7. Roast goose or roast duck
8. Smoked eel (not a bad dish—if you like it)
9. Natural cheese (most varieties)
10. Layer cake with frosting (only rich, deluxe varieties)
11. Liver sausage (best quality)
12. Peanut butter
13. Smoked ham (premium brand)
14. Caviar (I just put this in for fun! The calories are correct, but unfortunately the price isn't!)

So, if we think ahead, use every means available to us, and concentrate on the basic idea of getting maximum caloric mileage out of everything we eat, we will win. And we will be delighted to know that we can gain weight no matter where we eat—at home, take-out, restaurant, or microwave at work.

## Chapter Eight

# The Truth:
# More Pounds
# Mean Better Sex

**D**ebbie was the typical Glamour Girl. At 28 years old, with her long, blonde hair done up in a ponytail, upturned nose, bright blue eyes, and a perfect tawny skin, she looked like a model for a swimsuit commercial. From the neck up, that is. Debbie was 5 feet 6 and weighed 109 pounds. That gave her a Body Mass Index of 17.7—decidedly underweight. There was no swimsuit in the world that would make her feel right. That's what she was saying that afternoon in my office:

"Doctor, I have everything! I own three florist shops, I have my own condominium, I have a beach house and a sailboat. But I dread going to the beach and I never use my sailboat. I don't have to tell you why. For the beach you need a bathing suit—and to go sailing everyone I know wears shorts. At 109 pounds I'm not going to put on shorts and I'm afraid to buy a bathing suit. I can't even find a decent pair of jeans! Do you know why I want to gain weight?"

"Why?"

"Well, it's not just to go sailing. Let me tell you what happened last Saturday. I went to a club with Kelly, a girlfriend of mine. We were sitting at a table toward the back having a drink and these two nice-looking fellows came over to ask us to dance. The one that asked me was well dressed and well mannered. You know, different from the fellows you usually meet in places like that. He came up to our table and said: 'I hope I'm not intruding but if you'd like to dance with me, I'd be delighted.' That's a big improvement over the usual: 'Hey, Babe! What about it?'

"They were playing reggae and so we danced apart for a couple of sets. It turned out that he was an Assistant District Attorney and a really interesting person. Then they played a slow dance and when he took me in his arms, everything changed."

"What do you mean?"

Debbie shrugged. "Well, he got kind of nervous and then he said, 'Listen, have you been sick or something? I mean if you want to sit down and rest, it's okay with me.' "

Debbie's face flushed. "You know, that's the problem. As soon as he put his arms around me he realized that I'm skinny! Men want girls with bazooms and, you know, butts . . . something substantial! I don't blame him, but I have to do something about it!''

Debbie made an important point. Neither men nor women have to fit a predetermined stereotype as far as appearance is concerned, but we have to face the fact that we live in a world of expectations and anticipations. We should be able to explain to every potential male or female friend that body weight and contour are not that important. We should be able to make them understand that they should look beyond physical characteristics to discover our true value as a person. But most of the time we never get that opportunity.

Like it or not, this is a world of "first impressions." We are constantly compared with the ideal bodies we are shown on television, in films, in magazines, and everywhere else. Although there aren't enough pages in this book to change the world, there are more than enough to help us gain weight and change *ourselves*. Obviously the number-one reason for gaining weight is to improve our health and save ourselves from a premature death. Remember that underweight people die long before their time. But if at the same time and at no extra cost we can also improve our sexual attractiveness and our sexual performance (yes, that's right!) why not take advantage of the opportunity?

Here's the problem. Human beings, from a very early age, are imprinted with a preprogrammed image of what is sexually attractive. It varies somewhat from society to society but in general it works out to this:

A sexually attractive woman is supposed to have well-rounded curves—that is, enlarged breasts, rounded prominent buttocks, prominent calves of her legs, thighs that are well demarcated, and the absence of bony prominences. Specifically, her hip bones shouldn't stick out, her collarbones shouldn't protrude, and her shoulders should have a rounded and smooth appearance.

All of those characteristics come from one basic attribute: subcutaneous fat deposits. Human skin is made up of several layers. The top layer is called the "epidermis" and that's what we wear on the outside. Underneath is the next layer, called the "dermis." The dermis is full of little globules of fat—surrounded by fibrous tissue to hold them more or less in place. In women, after they start producing quantities of female sex hormones, the fat is deposited around their bodies according to a very specific plan. It goes to the buttocks and the hips to give them their characteristic rounded appearance. It goes to the breasts—especially the front part of the breasts—to make them stand out from the chest wall. The fat is also deposited all over the woman's body under the skin so that her silhouette is made up of smooth curves instead of the sharp angles that men's bodies have.

Fortunately, that's one of the real fringe benefits of gaining weight. As soon as a woman begins to put on weight, it goes straight to her hips, buttocks, and breasts. Remember the old lament of our *overweight* friends: "Two minutes on the lips, ten years on the hips!"

As usual, what is bad news for them is good news for us. For us, it may take a little longer than "two minutes on the lips," but you can be sure whatever we gain goes straight to the hips—and the breasts and the buttocks.

That's good news, but there is even better news than that. In some cases by utilizing a carefully chosen exercise we can make some of the fat deposits go where we want them even faster. Does that sound like too good to be true? Well, here's one exciting example.

If we stop to think about it scientifically, weight gain can be summed up in one technical word: "thermodynamics." It's a specialized word but what it means is "the movement or transfer of heat." Remember, a calorie is simply a measurement of heat. When we eat, we are transferring heat into our bodies and storing it in the form of fat. Then when we move around or exercise, we transform that fat into heat or energy to move our muscles. If the heat is enough to become noticeable, our body temperature rises, and we sweat.

Now, if we could only control that storage-of-heat-as-fat, we could deposit that fat in the places we wanted to see it the most. For example, in the case of Debbie, she could direct the fat deposits to what she charmingly called her "bazooms." But how? How can we do it?

Well, the seals do it. And if we take a cue from them, we can do it, too. Seals—especially those in northern climates—swim in cold water. To protect their vital organs from the cold, Nature has arranged for them to develop deposits of fat over the front part of their bodies. As a matter of fact, the whole underside of the seal is covered with a nice uniform layer of fat. And the colder the climate and the colder the water, the thicker the fat layer.

Can we do the same thing? Well, we don't want to plunge into frigid waters and swim for hours like the seals do. But we don't have to. It turns out that human beings are even more sensitive than seals to the effect of low temperatures on the front side of their bodies. Have you noticed that champion female swimmers are always a little "chunky" around the front? It's not just the exercise that causes it. It's the constant action of cool water on the front of their bodies as they swim.

How can we take advantage of that thermodynamic effect? It's easy. All we have to do is swim, just like the seals do. But we should look for a pool or a lake or a beach with cool water. It doesn't have to be polar bear temperature but about 72 to 74 degrees Fahrenheit is ideal. If you swim for 15 minutes a day in water of that temperature—and follow the Quick Weight-Gain Program—in less than 2 weeks you should notice increased fat deposits in your breasts and abdomen. Don't worry about the abdominal fat deposits. They won't give you a pot belly. The layer of fat should be thin and uniform and fit firmly between the abdominal muscles (rectus abdominus) and the dermis of your skin. It will give you smooth, attractive contours—just the way you like them. At the same time it will increase the fat deposits on your breasts. Here's a strange, but scientifically sound, point. Ideally you should do your swimming without any clothes on—just like the seals. That makes for uniform deposits of fat. There is no insulation from a bra or a swimsuit bottom. But since that's not always possible, just wear the briefest swimsuit that the circumstances will allow.

Men can do the same thing but with a word of caution. Men—with rare exceptions—don't usually deposit fat on the buttocks or breasts. (At least, not until they are well on their way to being seriously overweight.) Because of their male hormones (testosterone) their fat is directed to the abdominal area first. The explanation is—presumably—that abdominal fat is more available for immediate use in case of running, fighting, etc. Female fat deposits in the hips, breasts, and buttocks are thought to be more stable and serve as a suitable reserve for pregnancy and lactation. When we hear our overweight female friends complain about how hard it is to lose weight from the hips and buttocks, we can believe that explanation.

In any event, taking advantage of the "seal effect" to put weight on the abdomen can be a two-edged sword for men. It's a good idea to do it carefully and monitor your progress. One solution is for men to swim in warmer water—say 78 to 80 degrees—and keep a close eye on the rate of fat deposit until they reach the desired proportions.

But both men and women can do much more than just use swimming to direct bulk where they want it to go. Remember the exercises we mentioned in chapter 5? Well, that was just the beginning. There are some excellent exercises that will help you fill out your body wherever you feel you need it the most. But a word of caution!

If we want to put on weight, the basic principle is: "Fat is our friend." Now, that sounds too simple, doesn't it? Of course fat is our friend. But in more ways than one. You see, fat doesn't make any demands on you. It just sits there making your body look full and healthy.

Muscle is an entirely different story. Muscle is constantly metabolizing and using up energy. That means a certain proportion of whatever you eat goes to maintain your muscle. To put it another way, if you just sit around before you start on a program of muscle building, you will consume the familiar 1.5 calories a minute. But if you really develop a lot of muscles, you may increase your caloric "burn rate." Added fat doesn't burn more calories—but added muscle does.

Now, generally it's not much of a problem if you keep your exercise and muscle building within reasonable limits, at least at the beginning. Developing a big muscle mass that will devour calories is only really a problem for dedicated body-builders. But you should know about it. Now, as our English friends say, "Having said that," let's move on to moderate, carefully controlled muscle building to mold our bodies the way we want them.

Men who are underweight often want to have better-developed shoulders to fill out shirts and suits—not to mention looking better at the beach. The truth is, of course, that adding fat doesn't really do much for the shoulders, so a few shoulder-building exercises are certainly justified. By the way, whenever the subject of exercise comes up, I always look for a program that doesn't require any new clothes, new shoes, or new equipment. I always remember what Henry David Thoreau, the distinguished American philosopher, used to say: "Beware of all enterprises that require new clothes."

This one, like all the exercises here, doesn't require any clothes or new equipment or even new shoes. I especially like this one.

Lie on the floor on your back. Hold a can—a soup can will do fine or a book or a 1-pound weight—in each hand. Place both hands with the cans on your chest. Then stretch your hands back over your head but don't let the cans touch the floor. Count to 5 while you hold the cans over your head. Then slowly bring the cans back to their original position on your chest. Do it about 3 to 5 times to begin with, then gradually increase until you are doing about 15 repetitions a day.

You should begin to see a difference in about a week. In 4 weeks of daily repetitions, most people will have a nice increase in their shoulder development.

I mention soup cans or books because almost everyone has them around the house and all you need is something with weight. As you proceed you can add slightly heavier books or cans. If you already have store-bought weights, you can of course use them. Start with the light ones—say a pound or so—and increase them according to your comfort level. But don't overdo it or strain. The idea is moderate and gradual development of the target muscles. If it hurts or feels uncomfortable, *stop.*

Maybe this is a good time to repeat the standard type of warning that seems to appear everywhere these days: "Do not attempt a weight-gaining program unless and until you have had a thorough examination and consultation with your physician. If at any time during that program you experience any discomfort or serious symptoms, consult your physician immediately. If you experience any pain or discomfort during any exercises, stop immediately and consult your physician."

I know what you're thinking. "Why do I have to go to a doctor just to eat better and put on the weight I so desperately need?" The answer is that maybe you are underweight because of some physical condition that you don't know about yet.

Your next question might well be: "Why should I go to the doctor if all I'm going to do is lift a couple of soup cans or books—something I do every day anyhow?"

The answer is this: Don't go to the doctor just because you're going to lift a couple of soup cans. But if the lifting seems to cause you unusual discomfort, you should check with your doctor, of course. Common sense, right?

Now let's see some more exercises to help us fill out and firm up where we most want to fill out and firm up. How about a more advanced exercise to add bulk to the shoulders? Once you can do the previous shoulder exercise easily, try this one:

Lie on the floor on your back. Hold a can—just like before—in each hand. (The purpose of the cans is only to add weight and make the muscles work harder. Our muscles have little sensors built into them. When we make them work hard, they respond by automatically adding more fibers so they can lift more weight. More fibers add more bulk or volume to the muscle.) Place both hands with the cans on your chest. Then push the cans straight upward. When they are as high as they can go, let your hands drop back slowly over your head, but don't let the cans touch the floor behind your head. At that point your hands with the cans will be stretched over your head about 2 to 3 inches off the floor. Hold that position for a count of 10.

Then raise the cans over your head again and slowly lower them onto your chest. Do this 3 to 5 times to start, gradually increasing to 10 to 15 repetitions.

Both these exercises will build up your shoulder muscles very nicely. Don't underestimate them—they are very effective, and don't overdo them—they are very powerful exercises.

While shoulder development is most sought after by men, women can do these same exercises if they want to. They're especially nice if you like to wear strapless or off-the-shoulder outfits and want lovely curvaceous shoulders.

Another of the areas where underweight folks sometimes feel the lack of volume is the upper arms. The truth is that it's hard to deposit fat there quickly. But you can add muscle fairly easily with this routine:

Stand comfortably. Grab your cans again and hold them up at shoulder level on both sides of your body. Slowly raise them straight up above your head and hold them there for the count of 5. Then lower them slowly and rest for the count of 2. Then repeat the exercise 5 times. Gradually increase to 15 repetitions. You can also use heavier cans as you go along—or small weights. When the cans or weights you are using seem light to you, use something heavier.

Another superb upper arm exercise is this one: Grasp your books or cans or weights (one of my patients used *firm* cantaloupes in season) in each hand and hold them at waist level in front of you with your elbows loosely against your sides. Then raise your elbows like a bird flapping its wings while keeping your hands at least a foot apart. Hold that position for 1 second and go back to the original position slowly. Try 5 at first, gradually increasing to 15—but increase the number of repetitions very slowly. This is a powerful exercise, as you will see!

As they begin to gain weight, many women like to develop the calves of their legs. The rounded contour is very attractive and goes well with their new filled-out look. The calf muscle is called the "gastrocnemius," and is an easy one to develop. Try this:

Look for a shelf or counter or tabletop at about waist height that is too heavy for you to lift. Stand facing it and put the palms of both hands under it as if you were going to lift it. Push upward hard with both hands and at the same time stand up on your tiptoes. Hold that for the count of 3. Then let your heels drop until you are standing flat on the floor again. Repeat the exercise 5 times, gradually increasing it to 15 repetitions. But again, this is a power exercise, so go slowly and take it easy!

By the way, there's one important detail to keep in mind about any form of exercise while we are trying to gain weight. We shouldn't exercise—if we can manage our schedule that way—for an hour before eating or for an hour after eating. Why? Well, we don't want to empty the glycogen stores in the liver. Remember the story of glycogen? If we have calories stockpiled in the liver as glycogen, and our very limited glycogen storage space is all filled up, the carbohydrates and fat that we eat are directly deposited as fat. But if we exercise immediately after eating we dump the glycogen into our bloodstream, where it is used to supply energy to our actively contracting muscles. Then the food that we consume is diverted to replace the used-up glycogen in our liver. The same thing happens if we exercise just before eating. We leave room in our liver for more glycogen, and the digested food goes there first rather than being deposited as fat.

It's amazing how an understanding of some of the little-known scientific secrets of the human body can give us a tremendous advantage in our weight-gain program. With that in mind, what's the best time to exercise? Interestingly enough, the ideal time is at bedtime—just before going to sleep. During the night our metabolism is going to be at its lowest anyhow, so it doesn't matter if we deplete our glycogen stores. Nothing much is going to happen while we are asleep that will affect our weight-gaining project. And with a little extra exercise at bedtime, we will sleep much better.

What if you don't feel like exercising at bedtime? That's okay. Do it when you feel like it and when you can. But if you can avoid all physical activity for an hour before eating and for an hour after eating, you will give yourself an extra advantage in reaching your goal.

Let's look at some more exercises that will give us just the contours that we want. Developing the calves is useful and important, but many women express interest in developing their thigh muscles as well. After all, once they begin to put on weight, they are eager to get into swimsuits and go to the beach. But these days—as we've all seen—swimsuits emphasize the thighs. However, there's a minor problem in trying to add volume to the thighs. Almost all the exercises you see in exercise guides involve squatting. That is, they suggest you stand straight and then squat in place. As you stand up, the thigh muscles have to raise the entire weight of your body, and with enough repetitions, you will add mass in your thighs. And you will probably also add chronic low back pain to your life, not to mention knees that will forever let you know in advance when it's going to rain. Opening and closing your knees like a jackknife and squashing your vertebrae up and down won't do you any good in the long run. It's better not to round out your thighs if it's going to give you arthritis for the rest of your life.

Does that mean we have to suffer with thin thighs even though we put on weight everywhere else? Hardly. Here's a safe and simple exercise that will build thigh bulk and won't even come near your knees or your back. Here's the way it works:

Take a nice-size book—say about 9 to 10 inches high. Wrap it in a bath towel to soften the sharp edges. Sit down on a comfortable straight chair—a kitchen chair will do. Place the book between your knees the long way and hold it there by gently squeezing your knees together. Your knees should be about 9 to 10 inches apart. Then hold the book with both hands and squeeze it with your knees as hard as you can. Hold for 5 seconds and relax. Then squeeze it again. Do that for the usual 5 repetitions and gradually build it up to 15 repetitions. Try holding the book with only one hand so you can feel how hard your thigh muscles are contracting. This is a powerful exercise and one that leaves your knees and back alone. You'll like it.

Now, there's one exercise that appeals to everyone—men and women. The reason for that is it builds up one of the body's major visual "target" areas. A visual target area is what the rest of the world sees first when you walk into a room. Check it out yourself. The next time you are at a party or a meeting and someone enters the room, observe what part of their body most of the people look at first.

In most cases, it will be their face. That's essential to identify them, and once our weight-gain program takes hold, your face will be nicely filled out. The next area that most people look at is the part of your body from the shoulders to twelve inches below. That's the way you measure the size and muscular development of a man—and the breast size and development of a woman. (Don't blame me—I didn't devise this arrangement. It's just what people do by instinct.) So one of the most useful things we can do as part of our put-on-pounds program is fill out this key visual target area.

If we can add bulk to our chest we can greatly improve the appearance of this area in men as we gain weight—especially in proportion to the rest of our body. We can accomplish exactly the same thing in women—with one added advantage. We can make the breasts look bigger. Remember, breasts are mostly fat plus milk-producing glands. Their size is primarily determined by those "twin H's": Heredity and hormones, although gaining weight adds fat to the breasts and truly makes them bigger. But exercise can only develop muscle, and there is no "breast muscle" as such. But there are some muscles right under the breasts—and as we mentioned before, if we can develop those, they will push the breasts up and out. That will do more than the most expensive bra—and it will be 100 percent natural. Even better, when you take off your bra, the benefit won't evaporate.

The muscles that we want most to enlarge are the pectoralis muscles—the ones that lie on the front of the chest. The first exercise is an easy one to do, but it really packs a punch. You will feel the difference in a week or so. Here's the technique:

Stand with your back against a flat surface about waist high— more or less. The kitchen counter is ideal. Place both your hands at your sides on top of the counter. Then push down on the counter with both palms and raise your body until you're standing on your tiptoes. But here is the secret—don't raise yourself by pulling up your heels. Let your chest muscles do all the work—that's the way they will enlarge. This exercise is really superb for developing your chest. Why? Because you are using the muscles of your chest to raise your entire body weight. If you weigh 100 pounds, you are lifting 100 pounds.

But here is another point to watch. The height of the counter is critical. Try it first with one hand on the counter and the other hand feeling the muscles of your chest. If you feel the muscles tighten when you push yourself up, the counter is the right height. If you don't feel the muscles contracting fully, look for another counter either higher or lower. Do the usual 5 repetitions, raising it gradually to 15 repetitions as you improve.

The next exercise is another excellent one for pushing the breasts up and out and increasing their apparent size. It also develops the male chest so fast that before you know it you will have to buy bigger shirts. All you have to do is follow the instructions precisely and you will be amazed and delighted. Here we go:

First, find a reclining chair, a rocking chair, or a secretarial chair with a back that goes backward if you lean against it. If you don't have any of these handy, an easy chair or sofa will do. Sit in the chair or on the couch and lean back so you are half reclining and half sitting up. Your upper body should be at about a 45-degree angle. It's more or less the way people slump backward in their chairs when they have eaten much too much at Thanksgiving dinner.

Then take those trusty soup cans—or 1-pound weights—one in each hand. Raise the weights directly above your head and lower them slowly to shoulder height. But here's the key point: keep your elbows as far back as you can and bring the weights all the way down to shoulder height each time. Your hands should be facing forward. Keep your eyes on the ceiling while you are doing it and you will feel the muscles contracting just the way you want them to. Another useful tip: At every session, change the angle of your body just a little bit. Move your upper body a little forward or a little backward before you start. That will vary the angle of motion of your chest muscles and assure that they develop to the maximum. Do the usual 5 repetitions, raising it gradually to 15 repetitions as you proceed.

These exercises should supplement our weight gain very nicely. They provide extra bulk for arms, chest, breasts, thighs, and calves. When we add that to the weight we are gaining, we should have just the perfect body contours that we are seeking. It's easy, it's fun, and every day it brings us closer and closer to our goal.

## Chapter Nine

# Seventeen Secrets for Putting on Pounds Fast

**W**henever we think about hunger, we think about eating. And whenever we think about eating, we think about hunger. The truth is that most people only think about food when they *are* hungry. For those of us who are underweight, that's about it. We get hungry and we decide to eat. The other side of the coin—and the one that can make it harder to reach our goal—is this: If we're *not* hungry, usually we *don't* eat.

On the other hand, our overweight friends do just the opposite. They can eat *anytime*—and they usually do. They eat when they're worried, they eat when they're tense—usually more than under normal conditions. They even get up at night to eat all the things they haven't had a chance to eat during the day. They eat when they *are* hungry and they eat when they're *not* hungry. They just munch their way through life—gaining more and more weight as each day goes by.

What is their secret? What can we learn from them that will help us to gain weight? We don't want to get fat, but we want to gain weight. Can our overweight friends teach us anything useful?

I think so. If we want to gain weight we have to change our entire attitude about food. We have to make eating our number-one goal in life. After all, that's what most of the other people in this world think about—where their next meal is coming from and what they are going to eat. We need to break the pattern of only eating when we are hungry—the feeling of hunger may be very elusive in those of us who are underweight.

Think instead of eating whenever the opportunity arises. If you have a coffee break on the job, don't waste the opportunity just on a calorie-poor cup of coffee. At least have a sweet roll or a cupcake—a few cookies or some doughnuts. Eat something that will put a hundred calories or so under your belt. Doughnuts and coffee are especially good since the average doughnut will give you about 100 very useful calories.

Get into the habit of carrying something to eat with you—in your pocket or purse. It can be a couple of cookies wrapped in plastic or a doughnut or a little piece of cake or whatever treat most appeals to you.

If you like cookies, chocolate-covered peanut-butter cookies will give you about 120 calories each while those half-round marshmallow cookies covered with chocolate are good for almost 140 calories. Check out the cookie section in your supermarket, find the ones that appeal to you most, look for the highest caloric content, and carry a couple with you wherever you go.

It's a good idea to almost always eat at least three times a day—no matter what. Eat a nice breakfast, eat a good lunch, and eat a full supper. What if you just can't eat all that much? Then eat what you can. Make up your meals from the menus in chapters 14 and 15—or design your own. If you can't eat it all, eat as much as you can eat. But remember, try to finish within the magic 13 minutes before the cholecystokinin effect starts to shut down your appetite. Set the table, serve the food, and sit down to eat as if it were the most important thing in your life. (As a matter of fact, it is!)

As you go through your daily routine, look for small "eating adventures." If you pass a bakery that is just pulling freshly baked rolls out of the oven, stop in and have one or two. If a new place opens up in your neighborhood with freshly made sandwiches—heroes or submarines or torpedoes or whatever they may call them—drop in and try one. They probably won't ever be fresher than that first day!

Remember the old saying, *"Some people live to eat while others eat to live''*? The usual interpretation is that overweight people "live to eat" since food is always uppermost in their minds. On the other hand, underweight folks like us "eat to live," only consuming enough to keep our bodies working. But there's an entirely different meaning that goes beyond the original triteness of the saying. If we only "ate to live" before we realized how mortally dangerous underweight is, now we are committed to "eat to live" to literally *save our lives.*

One of the most helpful things you can do to accomplish that is to make food a part of your life. You must have noticed that most underweight folks don't really have much interest in food. They don't think much about how it is prepared, what it contains, and all the different nuances and possible combinations. To many of them, food is food. A cheese sandwich or a Duck à l'Orange is about the same. It's something to kill their hunger and get them back to what they were doing before. That was Beth's problem—at least in the beginning.

Beth is 31 and a lingerie designer, or as she puts it, "I'm into ladies' underwear!" She is 5 feet 7 and used to weigh 104 pounds, which gave her a B.M.I. of only 16.35—definitely underweight. Now she weighs 111 pounds. That gives her a Body Mass Index of 17.45. She's almost at the weight she finally aspires to—115 pounds. She has two outstanding qualities that have helped her a lot. She is determined—and she has a sense of humor.

"Look, Doctor, can you imagine how I felt? I used to spend all day designing these exciting undies for women about my age. I was drawing brassieres with nice big cups and deep vees so they could let their nice big round breasts hang right out. And when I got home from the office and started to change my clothes and looked in the mirror—what did *I* have?"

I had to smile.

"I don't know, Beth. What *did* you have?"

"Well, Doctor, you've seen those ads for the breast enlargers that they have on the back pages of some of those women's magazines? You've seen the 'Before' and 'After' pictures? The 'Before' is as flat-chested as the top of your desk, and the 'After' looks like she could float up to the ceiling, and if the wind was right, fly across Texas? Well, I wasn't 'Before' and I wasn't 'After.' I looked more like 'During.' You know I had something there and I was just hoping that some miracle would happen to make them grow.''

''And?''

''And it happened. After about a week on the Quick Weight-Gain Program I started to get this dull ache in my back—every time I would lean over the drawing board, I'd get a pain back there. After the third time I realized it was my bra getting tight! It worked, just like you said it would. But there was one thing that helped me above all. I want to tell you about it so you can pass it on to your other patients.''

''I'd like to hear it.''

Beth smiled. ''That's great! I know there are thousands of women out there just like me and if I can help them, it would be wonderful.

''Well, one thing that you said really struck a chord for me. You said, 'Get interested in food!' And the truth is that most of my life I never cared about food at all. I just ate what was there. If I went out to a restaurant, I always waited until someone else ordered and I said, 'I'll take the same!' But then I realized something very important.''

''What was that?''

''My success in the design world came from one thing. It's not that I'm so talented but I'm *determined.* I live and breathe fashion design. I read and study and look at everything I can find about fashion and design. I decided to do the same sort of thing about food. I started by watching some of those cooking shows on TV and reading some cookbooks. That was interesting but to tell you the truth, there was a problem.''

''What kind of problem, Beth?''

''I guess it's just me, but it wasn't stimulating enough. So I tried a different approach. Dan, my boyfriend, suggested we eat at a different kind of restaurant every week. You know, Thai one time and Moroccan another time and then Brazilian the next time. Fortunately there are a lot of these new ethnic restaurants these days. I was a little cautious at first—I didn't know what was going to happen.''

''How did it work out?''

''I couldn't believe it! It was so exciting! I suddenly discovered that there was life beyond hamburgers and pizzas! And there's something about ethnic food that makes you want to eat. I guess it's that whole rainbow of different colors and tastes and textures. I mean, the first bite you're not exactly sure. So you try it again. And then another bite. And then, wow! You're on your way!

''I think one of the reasons I wasn't eating enough was that my diet was so boring! But not now! And then Danny and I started trying out the recipes at home ourselves. It was a whole new world! We had to reach out beyond the supermarkets to find the ingredients and we met a whole new group of people and cultures that we didn't even know existed in this country. Have you ever eaten Lumpia, Doctor?''

Beth was so enthusiastic she didn't even wait for me to answer. ''It's wonderful! It's the Filipino version of Chinese egg roll but better! It's part Chinese and part Malay and it's sensational! You can fill it with almost anything and it tastes just as good cold as hot and it's even better the next day! It's the easiest thing in the world to make, and for 'enhancing,' there's nothing like it. You can put an extra 500 calories into it and you won't even know that they're there! Would you like the recipe, Doctor?''

You can see that Beth's excitement was contagious, and she was right on the target. Try new foods, try ethnic foods, try exciting foods. Remember that almost all of us have an ethnic cuisine in our background. Even the folks who came over on the Mayflower had some very special dishes that they brought with them. We'll see a lot more about ethnic dishes in chapter 10, and I'm sure you'll find them fascinating and very useful.

Another weapon that we can add to our weight-gaining arsenal is ''eating breaks.'' It's simple and painless and yet it adds important amounts of calories every 24 hours—calories that add up during the weeks and months to put on pounds effortlessly. Here's how it works:

Think of all the times during the day that you break from your daily routine to do something else. For example, you may take off ten minutes in the morning to check the latest salesman's reports or to review incoming financial news. You may go from the sales floor to the stockroom to check the merchandise. As soon as you change your daily rhythm, take advantage of the change of pace to nibble on something to eat. That's another habit of our overweight friends that we can very successfully adopt. I'm sure you've noticed: ''Fat people are *always* eating.'' Our problem is the opposite. How many times do our friends say, ''But I never see you eating! No wonder you're so thin!'' Well, from now on, let them see us eating—whenever we get the chance.

If you have a long commuting drive to and from work, be sure to pack something tasty to munch on along the way. It takes the monotony out of the trip and packs in the nourishment that we so badly need. What should it be? For drive time, you want something easy to manage, not overly spillable, and something that won't distract you from what's happening on the road ahead. Some good possibilities are any kind of cookie or wrapped pastry snacks like sweet rolls, doughnuts, or brownies. You can also munch on dried fruit, nuts, raisins, and things like that. By the way, if you like macadamia nuts, you're in luck. A mere ounce of those delicious little spheres will add over 200 calories to your daily intake. Peanuts aren't so bad either—and much cheaper. An ounce of those will add about 180 calories. Try always to have something to eat in your car—for drive time and emergencies.

Emergencies? Is there such a thing as a ''weight-gain emergency''? If we think about it, there is. There are only 24 hours in a day, each hour with 60 minutes. As we have seen, during every one of those 1,440 minutes—even when we are asleep—we are losing a minimum of 1.5 calories just to keep alive. When we walk, run, swim, dance, or do chores, we burn up much more than that. If we are underweight and we miss a meal—or an opportunity to eat—we lose a chance that will never come again. Never in that day, never in that year, never in our entire lives. Think about it.

Many years ago I was at a graduation ceremony at a large university. The speaker, a very wise and distinguished gentleman, gave a very short and right-to-the-point graduation speech. Basically he said this:

Most of you who are graduating are about 22 years old. If you live to be 72—which I hope all of you will—you will see 2,600 weeks go by. If you read one book a week—every week for the rest of your life—you will only learn what is in 2,600 books. That is barely enough to prepare you to deal with all the challenges of a very complex and demanding society. I suggest you start reading *today*—and never stop.

That was excellent advice and I recommend it to everyone. But it's also excellent advice when it comes to gaining weight. We only have so many hours in the day to eat—and when they are gone, the opportunity will *never* return. If we miss breakfast, that's it. You can't eat breakfast at noon because then it's lunchtime. And you can't eat lunch at 6:00 P.M. because that's dinner time. So what happens if for some reason you get up late and have to rush off to work without breakfast? If you miss the meal completely, you will be down at least 1,000 calories for the day. Your body burns up those 1,000 calories in 11 hours. If you miss breakfast, you've lost 11 hours of vital caloric value—*forever.* But there's a solution. Even if you rush out, jump into your car, shoot out the driveway, and get on the road, you haven't lost your chance.

You can just settle back, put some nice music on the car stereo, and reach into your console. Take out a package of dried dates and start munching. If you consume just a cup of those tasty morsels, you will have rescued about 650 calories of that ''lost'' breakfast. Four nice cookies will add at least 250 more calories, and before you get to work you're up to 900 calories. Add a handful of peanuts, and you've replaced those missed calories. In these tense and overloaded days that kind of ''calorie emergency'' can come up almost anytime. Don't risk it!

Another excellent eating break is the television hour. This is the bane of our overweight colleagues. That's when the beer and potato chips and pretzels and pizza expand their waistlines. If only we could get the same results! But the good news is that we can!

Their problem—and our solution—is "unconscious eating." They complain that they can eat a whole bag of potato chips without even knowing it—when they become absorbed in an exciting program. And it's true. When they are totally involved in a thrilling movie, their hand moves automatically from the bag of snacks to their mouth and back again. It's the same with pizza or fried chicken or hamburgers. It's "Lift, bite, lower. Lift, bite, lower," and before they know it, it's 250 calories down the hatch. Wonderful! What's the secret? It's really the same secret as the one that guarantees a successful medical practice.

When I first opened my medical clinic, I was having coffee in the doctors' lounge at the hospital with an old practitioner. We were discussing the challenges of starting out in medicine. We talked of the various possibilities and finally he put down his coffee cup, looked me straight in the eye, and said, "Doctor, the key to success lies in two words—both ending in 'ability.' To be really successful, you need 10 percent *'ability'* and 90 percent *'availability'!'"

I don't know if he was right about that, but I do know that it applies precisely to gaining weight. If food is not available, you can't eat it. In the same way, if you have good high-calorie food at hand when you are watching TV, you are likely to eat it.

Try it tonight or tomorrow night. Make up a little tray of snacks and an open bottle of soda pop. Put it at your elbow and start to watch your favorite program. Open the bag of chips or the bag of dried fruit. Pour out the icy cold soda pop. *Start eating.* Take a bite or two, hold the bag in your hand, take a drink of the pop. The more interesting and exciting the program, the better. Forget about your diet, forget about your weight, forget about everything—just concentrate on eating and watching, eating and watching. If you do it right, you'll be amazed and delighted with the results.

You can do the same thing with pizza or a hamburger or fried chicken or whatever you like most. The key is to have the food at hand and to take the *first bite.* That starts the digestive reflexes and encourages you to eat more and more. But make sure it is something you like. If you like chocolate-chip ice cream, that's what it should be. If you like tortilla chips, put that on your tray. If a milk shake is your favorite, whip up a milk shake before you sit down to watch television.

The same technique works with the movies with certain exceptions. For some reason no one really knows, popcorn has become the traditional snack at the movies. It's interesting when you think about it. Why popcorn? And why only in the United States? Hot buttered popcorn is fine—or hot popcorn with whatever they put on it in the movies. But not necessarily for those of us who want to gain weight.

A cup of freshly popped popcorn is only about 45 calories and it fills you up fast! Even if you put a tablespoon of oil on it, you only get about 170 calories. And that's usually all you are going to eat for the 3 hours that a double feature takes. You're better off caloriewise taking your own snacks to the movies. The usual nuts, raisins, dried fruit, cookies, and other compact high-calorie goodies will do the job for you more efficiently. (Can you take fried chicken or hamburgers or pizza to the movies? Sure you can! If it's a Drive-In.)

So one of the basic principles of food management in our Quick Weight-Gain Program might be summed up as: "Never leave home without something to eat!" We need to constantly refill our calorie reservoir and we usually do it three times a day at meals. But if for some reason we can't eat at mealtime, we mustn't let that calorie-refilling moment go by. "Night and day, at home and away—always have food available."

Just a moment. Did we say "*night* and day . . ."? Do we need to have food available at *night*, too? Well, it isn't an absolute necessity but it would certainly be helpful. One of the secrets of overweight people is night eating. So many of them wake up at night to eat. They don't usually brag about it, but "raiding the refrigerator at midnight" is one of their most common ploys.

It's an interesting situation. Assume that the last meal was supper at 6:00 P.M. By 2:00 A.M. they have gone 8 hours without anything to eat. That's the longest period of time without nourishment in their entire 24-hour day. Even the space from lunch to supper is only 6 hours or so. If we analyze it, it's fair to assume that they could reasonably be hungry 2 hours after midnight. And for them, it's a problem. But for us, it's an advantage.

It may be too much to expect someone who is underweight to arise at 2:00 A.M. and trot downstairs to the fridge to polish off a ham sandwich, a piece of pie, and a dish of chocolate ice cream. That would simplify the job for everyone in short order. But there is a technique here that we can benefit from.

Most people get up at least once during the night—usually to urinate. (*I'm a doctor, so I can say the word.*) Few of us are eager—at that moment—to make the long pilgrimage to the kitchen, turn on the lights, open the refrigerator, take out the food, and settle down to eat. It takes a lot more internal pressure and compulsion to eat than most of us have at that particular moment. However, if we have a little snack available right at our bedside at the moment when we feel even the slightest pang of hunger, the opportunity to add a few hundred calories won't slip through our fingers.

What should we put aside for that midnight refill? For those lucky enough to have a small refrigerator in their bedroom they don't even have to choose. Anything that goes in the icebox will be fine. They can have ice cream, milk shakes, cheese, and anything else they might have a taste for. And sometimes you only feel like eating something that has to be refrigerated. For example, during some of those scorching summer nights when you really can't sleep only a nice dish of ice cream will do. But who wants to march into the kitchen, and go through the whole routine? But the taste for ice cream is on your tongue and the calories would be more than welcome. What do you do? Roll over and go back to sleep?

You don't have to. How about one of those nice little plastic cooler boxes right next to your bed? You know, the kind they sell at the sporting goods stores? Just pop a pint (or more if you like) of your favorite ice cream—and anything else that has to stay cool—in the insulated cooler along with a spoon. When you wake up during the night, you have everything you need right at the bedside. And here's the bonus. If you eat high-calorie food at night, you are almost sure to wake up heavier in the morning.

There's another fringe benefit too. If your spouse needs to gain weight too, both of you can enjoy the snack and have a little togetherness at the same time. Remember, there's no law against having fun—much less if you can gain weight in the process. And that brings up a very important point.

You can achieve your goal faster and easier if you can eat while you're having fun. Remember when we were discussing the Opioid Feeding Drive and the effect of cholecystokinin on our appetite? That's when we suggested taking eating seriously, in the sense of sitting down to eat and just eating. That was important because of the 13-minute limit to our appetite once the cholecystokinin secretion is triggered. That's certainly true and we have to constantly keep it in mind. But now that we understand that, there's another mechanism that we can use to make progress.

It's something you've seen many times and perhaps experienced on more than one occasion. It's what we call "socially promoted eating." Remember the last time you were on a picnic? Remember all that food that was laid out? It could have been a baked ham and fried chicken, hot dogs, hamburgers, maybe a lot of it barbecued, with a wonderful aroma and good feelings all around? There were a lot of people and everyone talking and socializing. And everyone eating. Eating while they talked, eating while they walked, eating standing up, eating sitting down, eating half lying on the ground. And the beauty of that situation is that no one even thinks of what they eat.

"Here, have another hot dog!"

"Try some of these barbecued ribs!"

"What do you mean, you're not going to try my cherry pie?"

"You've just *got* to try this luscious watermelon!"

Who can resist those offers? That's right, no one. And before you know it, you've put away a thousand calories or so. Take advantage of any happy social occasion to eat. Because of the emotions and the excitement, both the Opioid Feeding Drive and the Cholecystokinin Effect get pushed into the background.

What happens under those circumstances is the emotional push to eat takes over, and you can eat much more than you would ordinarily. Christmas, Thanksgiving, birthdays, anniversaries, New Year's, and almost any kind of party can supply the opportunity for socially promoted eating. Even football games with the "tailgate picnic" or baseball games can provide the background for extra calories with no extra effort.

As a matter of fact, socially promoted eating is one of the rare opportunities for underweight folks to eat like overweight people do. Think about it. Most of our overweight friends suffer from "emotional eating." When they are tense or depressed or anxious, they are pushed by their emotions to overeat. The emotional pressure is what takes the brakes off and makes them eat far more than they really need to.

Now, in our case, in exciting social situations, our emotions are stimulated and we are pushed by our surroundings to eat more—and without the normal Opioid Feeding Drive and cholecystokinin brakes to hold us back. Now, we don't have to be depressed or anxious or tense—and we shouldn't be. But we can ride the crest of the emotional wave to eat more—*and gain more*—than we would under the usual circumstances.

There's something else that can release those normal Opioid Feeding Drive and cholecystokinin brakes. But you have to know how to use it. If you do it right, it can help you to eat more without being held back.

The secret is to use alcoholic beverages to stimulate your appetite so that you can eat more. (By the way, if you don't drink, wanting to put on pounds is *not* the reason to start.) For reasons that no one understands, under certain circumstances some kinds of drinks can make you eat more. It might be the alcohol itself that short-circuits the secretion of cholecystokinin at the same time it intensifies the Opioid Feeding Drive. No one really knows at this stage, and the exact way it works isn't important right now. What is important is that it *does* work. That's the easy part.

The part that takes some work is discovering the combination that's right for us. Some people already know what works for them. The rest of us (if we already drink and want to use alcohol as an extra push) have to experiment carefully. One of the traditional drinks to stimulate the appetite—especially in Europe—has been the aperitif. This is usually a combination of various herbs, often described on the label as *"a secret mixture handed down through the years."* Some examples are Vermouth, DuBonnet, Amer Picon, and about 100 others. Almost all of them are a mixture of wine and various herbs.

Hundreds of years ago these mixtures were used as medicines. Doctors and hospitals were few and far between in the Europe of the 1600s. But every household had its wine—usually homemade. And every garden had its herbs—instead of the modern-day medicine chest. The trouble was that many of the herbs were bitter and sour and funny tasting. However, one of the easiest—and most palatable—ways to take these herbal combinations was to dissolve them in wine. (We do the same thing these days when we prescribe a cough medicine dissolved in an alcoholic liquid.)

Vermouth is a good example. It can have as many as 16 different herbal ingredients including cinnamon, clove, and coriander. It also contains nutmeg, quinine, and tansy—all powerful drugs in herbal form.

(Are you surprised that nutmeg is a powerful drug? As a matter of fact it is an *hallucinogenic* drug, if taken by the tablespoonfuls. That's why jails and mental hospitals keep the kitchen nutmeg under lock and key.) These days we get our medication from pills—and the aperitifs are just kept behind the bar. But specifically because of their medicinal herb content, sometimes they can help stimulate our appetite. Most of them have a bitter under-flavor and one of the possible explanations is that they stimulate the flow of gastric juices and thereby increase the appetite.

Now, no one can tell you which one—if any—will help you. It's just a matter of trial and error. If you like the idea and you want to try it, take an ounce or so—no more—about half an hour before mealtime and see what the results are. You should keep in mind that an aperitif makes some people hungrier and takes away the appetite of others. You have to experiment to see if it works for you. Since you are going to use so little and you are going to take it like medicine, get the very best quality. A few possibilities might be: Campari, DuBonnet, Amer Picon, Vermouth (only the very best quality, preferably French), Pernod, Byrrh, and Punt e Mes. You can try any of the dozens of others, but the basic quality is a bitter taste. If it works for you, fine. If not, you've had a whole new set of interesting experiences.

For most people, hard liquor like whiskey or gin before a meal doesn't do a lot for their appetite. However, if you like a drink now and then, it won't interfere with your diet and you may find that it improves your appetite and allows you to gain weight a bit faster. The caloric value of a 2-ounce cocktail, for example, varies all the way from about 130 calories for a dry martini to almost 200 calories for a Black Russian—coffee liqueur and vodka. A banana daiquiri will put about 180 calories under your belt—if you like the taste. (I am omitting the ingredients for this one. If you drink already you know the recipe. If you don't drink, this is *not* the combination to start off with.) An ounce and a half of drinks like whiskey, vodka, or gin will give you about 100 calories or so depending on the alcohol content. But *don't* take up drinking just to gain weight.

What about wine? It's the same situation as the aperitifs. If a small glass of wine before a meal improves your appetite and stimulates you to eat more, it's worthwhile. The wines most likely to help you are the dry white wines, although some people get hungrier with a medium-dry red wine. Probably one of the best possibilities is a few sips of the best French champagne before dinner. It has one big drawback, however. Although it might add bulk to your weight program, it will make your wallet rather emaciated.

Beer is the other alcoholic possibility. Many people find beer so filling that it interferes with their ability to eat calorie-rich food. Once again, it's a matter of individual taste. If you enjoy a beer with dinner and find you can eat a good full caloric meal, you won't interfere with your progress. But don't *start* to drink beer thinking that it will be an important part of your program.

That brings us to a very important—and controversial—area of weight gain. We've all seen weight lifters, football players, boxers, and other big-bulk athletes, and I'm sure we've wondered from time to time how they manage to gain that massive amount of weight and keep it on. Some of them do it by taking steroids. These are pills or injections of a drug that changes the function of their bodies so that the weight goes on quickly and easily. *But you shouldn't do it.* You shouldn't ever do it. Steroids are basically forms of male sex hormones—testosterone—or variations on that basic molecule. They put on weight by intensifying the buildup of tissue and slowing down the breakdown of tissue. In simple terms it works this way:

Within our bodies, two events are constantly occurring. One is called "catabolism," where older cells and tissues are broken down and excreted. At the same time, another process called "anabolism" is going on. That's where new cells and tissues are created from the basic building blocks of the food we eat. The steroids are really "anabolic" hormones that stimulate "anabolism" and deemphasize "catabolism." But being basically male-hormone oriented, they also can damage the liver, enlarge the prostate, cause atrophy of the testicles, and other disastrous side effects. They can also make the men who take them uncontrollably aggressive and disruptive. They are *not* a good way for a man to gain weight under any circumstance. And no woman should ever even think of taking steroids—unless she wants to turn her sex hormone balance topsy-turvy, and her life as well.

There is also another weight-gain hormone out there that we should know about. It's called "somatotropic hormone," or STH for short. This is the real "growth" hormone, secreted by the pituitary gland. It reduces the fat deposits of the body at the same time that it increases the development of muscle tissue. At first glance, that would seem to be a dream come true for those of us who want to gain weight. But like all other attempts to bypass Mother Nature, it has big problems as well. One of the really serious possible side effects is diabetes mellitus—often called "sugar diabetes" or "ordinary diabetes." (There is another kind of diabetes called "diabetes insipidus," also related to the pituitary gland—it's important to emphasize the difference.) What good is a perfect body if you have given yourself diabetes for life? STH is obviously *not* the answer for underweight.

That brings us to the important question: Is there any pill that we can take—safely—that will help us gain weight? Although it sounds too good to be true, there is one pill that might—*just might*—increase our appetite and help us to gain weight faster. And strangely enough, it's a mystery pill. No one knows how it works, why it works, and we can't even guarantee that it will work. But it's safe, inexpensive, and harmless. The pill is plain old thiamine, otherwise known as vitamin $B_1$, available at your local drugstore or even your supermarket. For some people, 10 milligrams of thiamine a day has an almost magical effect. After about 3 days, they notice a kind of gnawing hunger that impels them to eat more than before. Sometimes a regular meal doesn't satisfy them, and they look for snacks within an hour after eating. Not everyone has the same effect but *if* it works, the results are wonderful. Another possible effect is nighttime hunger. In the hour or so before going to sleep, many people who take thiamine feel a need to eat and eat. It's worth trying—and it just might give us that little extra push that would be so welcome.

But simple vitamin $B_1$ or thiamine is about as far as we want to go in the pill department. All the rest of the medications for weight gain are just too exotic or outright dangerous for us. The truth is, the Quick Weight-Gain Program is so simple, so safe, so effective—and so enjoyable—that there is no reason to even consider measures that are unsafe, unappetizing, or hazardous to your health. If we simply follow the diet calmly and with determination, we will see the pounds come back on, week after week after week.

## Chapter Ten

# How Vegetarians Can Gain Weight Easily: The Organoleptic Connection

**J**eff was tense, there was no doubt about it. He fidgeted in his chair, he looked around my office, then out the window. Nervously he leaned over to rearrange some papers on my desk. As the Manager of a large Metropolitan Air Terminal he was used to stress, but obviously something very important was on his mind.

"What's the trouble, Jeff? What can I do to help you?"

"I don't think anyone can help me, Doctor! I have one of those impossible dilemmas. I'm too thin—you can see that. But there's no way I can gain weight without ruining my life. And I'm desperate to gain weight!"

"How much do you weigh, Jeff?"

He winced. "One hundred thirty-two and a half. And I'm 5 feet 11¼. And that means I'm undeniably underweight!"

"There's no doubt about that, Jeff. Let's see, you have a Body Mass Index of 18.29. That's something to be concerned about, but I don't think that *desperate* is exactly the right word."

Jeff sighed. "No, *desperate* is the word that fits my situation, Doctor. Look, I know the hazards of underweight, I know it really puts my life at risk, I know that I have to gain weight as soon as possible. But I also know I can't do it! Ever!"

"But what makes you so sure? Have you tried to gain weight?"

Jeff smiled wryly. "I've been trying to put on weight for—let's see, I'm 35 now. I've been trying to gain for almost 8 years. But I can't put on weight, and I never will.''

"But why are you so pessimistic? What makes you so sure you can't do it?"

"Because I'm a vegetarian, that's why! There is no way that anyone can gain weight on a vegetarian diet. Be honest, Doctor. Have you ever seen a fat vegetarian?'' Jeff suddenly stiffened. "What are you smiling at? Do you find that funny?''

"No, that's not the reason I'm smiling. I'm smiling because your problem isn't nearly as serious as you think it is. Of course you can gain weight as a vegetarian! And as a matter of fact, you are going to gain weight on a vegetarian diet. I'll bet you can put on a pound or two before this week is over.''

"But what about all the thin vegetarians you see everywhere? Have you ever seen an overweight vegetarian?''

"Have you ever been to India? They have about 400 million vegetarians there and at least a couple of million of them are on the chubby side. Don't worry, you'll gain all the weight you want to gain.''

And of course, Jeff gained the weight. Here's how:

The biggest problem that vegetarians have in putting on weight is that of mixed goals. There are millions and millions of vegetarians in the United States—with hundreds more joining the ranks every day. In the world as a whole there are probably close to a billion non–meat eaters at any given moment. In this country most people become vegetarians for one of two reasons. The first is moral conviction. They don't believe in killing animals to eat. That's their decision, and we wouldn't even think of arguing with them. The other motivation is health. Many people believe that a vegetarian diet is healthier than a meat-based diet. That question is a very interesting one, but a bit beyond the scope of this book.

However, it is possible to combine the two goals—don't eat meat and yet gain weight—if we are ingenious, inventive, and flexible. (The only exception is the super-strict vegetarians who only eat foods of plant origin. They don't consume milk, eggs, cheese, or anything that comes from an animal. It's possible to help them gain weight, but it is a difficult task. It really requires a separate book just for them.)

How are we going to do it? Here's how. First we are going to have to delve a little bit into ethnic recipes because the traditional American and Western European diet tradition is based on meat, fish, and chicken—plus other types of poultry and seafood. But other cultures—older by far—have perfected high-calorie nonmeat staples.

Secondly we are going to have to enhance our menus energetically and enthusiastically. We are going to have to use a lot of new and interesting tricks to bring the calories up to the maximum and bring the tastes up to their peak.

But there's plenty of good news. It isn't going to be that hard. Because they eat differently, vegetarians are accustomed to modifying and improvising their menus and even doing some of their cooking themselves.

But first let's ask the key question. What was Jeff eating, and why wasn't he gaining weight? Here's the answer. This is the kind of breakfast he was having:

### TRADITIONAL BREAKFAST

6 ounces orange juice (frozen)—72 calories
1 egg (boiled)—82 calories
1 cup of cornflakes with 4 ounces milk—160 calories
1 piece of toast, with 1 tsp. butter (or margarine)—90 calories
1 cup of coffee, black—2 calories
*Total:* 406 calories

A typical vegetarian breakfast? Yes, but so is this one:

## QUICK WEIGHT-GAIN PROGRAM ENHANCED BREAKFAST

6 ounces bottled grape juice—122 calories

1 egg (fried)—108 calories

1 cup of Grape Nuts, with 4 ounces of Half & Half—
575 calories

1 English muffin, with 2 tablespoons butter (or margarine)—345 calories

1 cup of coffee, with 1 ounce of cream and sugar—100
calories

*Total:* 1,250 calories

Isn't that interesting? It's our old friend, the Quick Weight-Gain Program Enhanced Breakfast from chapter 6! We don't have to change anything at all, and we have a complete and perfect 1,250-calorie vegetarian breakfast. And it's a breakfast that's perfectly acceptable to almost every practicing vegetarian (except for the strictest of all who don't eat any eggs or dairy products; and as we mentioned, it's a whole separate project to help that very small group gain weight).

The truth is that most breakfasts are vegetarian breakfasts—except for the ones that have bacon or sausage or similar additions—and we can even find a way around that problem as well.

But now let's look into the basic concepts of the Vegetarian Weight-Gain Diet. The challenge is right there in front of us. We have to find something that will replace meat, fish, and poultry and yet supply the same amount of concentrated calories. Can we do it? Of course we can! Let's start out with a few simple facts.

Beef, pork, and lamb have, on the average, about 100 calories per ounce. Most common cheeses have, on the average, exactly the same number of calories. On the other hand, chicken (fried with the skin on) has only about 55 calories per ounce. Goose has the same number of calories as meat—more or less—but it's not a prominent item on most daily menus. Fish, in general, runs about 30 calories per ounce, so it's easy to substitute higher-calorie vegetarian foods for the fish that vegetarians don't eat.

Viewed from this perspective, all of a sudden designing and following a vegetarian-oriented Quick Weight-Gain Program doesn't look so hard. And of course, it's not hard. Let's start right off with a typical lunch:

### VEGETARIAN QUICK WEIGHT-GAIN PROGRAM
### AT-WORK LUNCH-BOX LUNCH

2 slices rye bread—182 calories

2 ounces sliced Swiss cheese—220 calories

3 tablespoons mayonnaise—300 calories

2 leaves lettuce—3 calories

¼ tomato, sliced—8 calories

4 ounces dates—376 calories

1 piece of cake (frozen devil's food from supermarket)—293 calories

1 tablespoon whipped cream on top of cake—50 calories

8 ounces lemon-lime canned fruit drink—128 calories

*Total:* 1,560 calories

By substituting Swiss cheese for the bacon we ended up with a Swiss cheese on rye sandwich and lost a mere 20 calories in the process. But then we added a bare 1 tablespoon of whipped cream on top of the cake and gained 50 calories. So our net caloric intake for the vegetarian version of the Quick Weight-Gain Program At-Work Lunch-Box Lunch is 1,560 calories, or 30 calories more than the meat-eating version! So being a vegetarian is no disadvantage in our weight-gain program. As we will see as we move along, it can even be a help.

Let's see how we can apply the same principles to a vegetarian supper. Here's the meat-eater's supper:

## QUICK WEIGHT-GAIN PROGRAM SUPPER

8-ounce bowl of soup (ready-to-serve canned split pea soup with ham)—186 calories

T-bone steak, untrimmed, ¼ pound with 1 tablespoon melted butter (or margarine) on steak—639 calories

Salad: ½ California avocado with 2 tablespoons bottled Italian dressing—350 calories

1 cup mashed potatoes, with milk and butter (or margarine) added—200 calories

½ cup green peas in butter sauce (frozen)—90 calories

½ cup cut green beans in mushroom sauce (frozen)—100 calories

1 crescent roll with 1 tablespoon butter (or margarine)—202 calories

Apple pie, 4-ounce slice—415 calories

*Total:* 2,182 calories

Now let's see the vegetarian version. Will it meet the calorie test?

## VEGETARIAN QUICK WEIGHT-GAIN PROGRAM SUPPER

8-ounce bowl of soup (cream of mushroom soup with milk)—217 calories

Cheese ravioli, 8 ounces—628 calories

Salad: ½ California avocado with 2 tablespoons bottled Italian dressing—350 calories

1 cup mashed potatoes, with milk and butter (or margarine) added—200 calories

½ cup green peas in butter sauce (frozen)—90 calories

½ cup cut green beans in mushroom sauce (frozen)—100 calories

1 crescent roll with 1 tablespoon butter (or margarine)—202 calories

Apple pie, 4-ounce slice—415 calories

*Total:* 2,202 calories

We've substituted mushroom soup for the ham and pea soup and gained 31 calories. We chose ravioli instead of steak and "lost" 11 calories in the process. But the vegetarians still come out ahead, for a net gain of 20 calories. Is that much? It sure is, when you consider that we are totally eliminating meat—an entire category of one of the highest calorie foods—from our menu. And we still end up calories ahead! With the Quick Weight-Gain Program anything is possible!

There is no doubt whatsoever that the Quick Weight-Gain Program is a simple, safe, and satisfying way for vegetarians to gain the weight they need. If we keep a few basic concepts in mind, nothing can hold us back. Let's start with grains.

One of the apparent problems—and we say "apparent" because there aren't any real problems that can stand up to the Quick Weight-Gain Program—that vegetarians face is that so much of their daily consumption is made up of grains. And grains, by definition, have a lot of fiber. So the first thing we have to do is lower the fiber content of the grains we eat.

But then, what happens to the "high-fiber" diet? I can answer that question because I am the "Godfather" of the high-fiber diet. I was the first person to introduce the high-fiber diet as we know it today and published the first book on that diet, *The Save-Your-Life Diet,* in 1975, as well as *The Save-Your-Life Diet High-Fiber Cook Book* (together with my wife). I understand the problem perfectly well. There is no better diet in the world than that one—but to achieve our goal we have to put it aside for a few months while we deal with the most urgent item on our personal agenda: gaining weight. We won't do ourselves any lasting harm if we eat a low-fiber diet for the short time it takes to get our weight back to normal. And then we can go back to high fiber all the way.

Let's start with a vegetarian favorite: rice. The typical brown or unpolished rice has about 3 times as much fiber as white rice. That means it fills you faster and keeps you full longer. But we can't tolerate getting full faster and staying full longer if we are on a weight-gaining program. So it's white rice for the duration of the program. And rice is a wonderful food for vegetarians—it opens up a whole new range of opportunities for caloric enhancement. Look at it like this:

One cup of cooked rice has about 185 calories. But we can easily add at least 3 tablespoons of oil to it before serving. That brings up the total calories to 560, and if we add 2 ounces of pignolia nuts to make Middle Eastern–type rice, we get a total of 912 calories in a mere cupful of an easy-to-make, delicious, flavorful rice dish. There are many more exciting vegetarian dishes in chapters 14 and 15. But the point is clear and obvious: we can eat well and gain weight on our vegetarian routine.

Another favorite among vegetarians is bulghour, or bulgur. This is a form of wheat that has been "cracked" and parboiled. It looks a little like rice and tastes like a cross between rice and wheat. There are dozens of appetizing recipes for bulgur dishes, including some that can be eaten cold as salads. (Wait until you see that one! It's unique and gives a whole new dimension to vegetarian eating!)

All the other vegetarian favorites easily harmonize with the Quick Weight-Gain Program. That includes such favorites as beans. The bean is a wonderful legume in that it can soak up amazing amounts of calories while adding flavor and body. A cupful of beans is about 240 calories. But if those same beans are mashed, flavored, enhanced, fried, and mixed with delicious globs of melted cheese, they pack an impressive caloric punch. One excellent method is the famous "refried beans" of Mexico. Spread a generous portion of piping-hot refried beans on a steaming tortilla, top with fresh white cheese, and you have a superb gourmet dish that will add extra pounds at the same time. Making refried beans is an art passed from one generation to the next. Your best bet is to buy a good brand of already prepared refried beans.

Garbanzo beans (also known as "chickpeas") are another special food item, neglected by most meat eaters and well known to most vegetarians. For anyone who wants to gain weight, they should be much better known, because a mere ½ cup of raw chickpeas gives us a big 360 calories. And there are a dozen ways of preparing garbanzos that make them more exciting than most people have ever imagined. For example, there is a garbanzo dip for chips that makes other dips pale by comparison when it comes to both flavor and calories.

There is a dynamite "fast-food" version of garbanzos that you can make at home and underweight children will line up for seconds and thirds. Another specialty that appeals to children and adults alike is roasted flavored chickpeas that you eat like peanuts. You can make them in barbecue, garlic, cheese, onion, or any other flavor. They are much cheaper than peanuts and offer a nice change. (By the way, you'll find some techniques for dealing with the problems of underweight children in chapter 11.)

Here's the recipe:

### Spicy Garbanzo Nuts
Drain the liquid from a can of garbanzo beans (the label may say "chickpeas"). Put the beans into a large bowl. Mix thoroughly with garlic powder or onion powder (or both) or barbecue spice mix. About a tablespoon is right for each can—but use your own judgment.

Spread beans on a cookie sheet one bean high and roast at 250 degrees for about one hour or until the beans are firm and dry. If you like them hard like nuts, roast longer but keep an eye on them after the first hour.

If you'd like to try a super-good dip made from garbanzos, here's a great recipe:

### Spicy Garbanzo Dip
Drain the liquid from a can of garbanzo beans. Put the beans in a food processor or blender and add the juice of 1 medium lemon, ½ teaspoon of garlic powder, a pinch of black pepper, and ½ cup of olive oil. Blend until completely smooth.

This is a great dip with crackers, potato chips, or you can even spread it on hot pita bread.

It also opens the door to another excellent weight-gaining opportunity. Try this:

## FALAFEL ON PITA

Follow the same recipe but only add ¼ cup of olive oil to the seasoned beans. Process until smooth and then drop by the tablespoonful into hot olive oil. When cooked to the point of firmness, scoop out with a slotted spoon and drop into a pocket of hot pita bread.

As long as we are talking about vegetarian recipes, it's interesting to note that more than half the people in the entire world are vegetarians. For most of them, it's by choice. It's not that they are too poor to afford meat dishes. It's a matter of religious conviction among Buddhists and Hindus and a question of cultural traditions and tastes for most of the rest.

That's excellent news for vegetarians everywhere, because it means that we have literally thousands of tried-and-true mouth-watering recipes to choose from. But the news is even better than that. Because of the tremendous popularity of ethnic and regional cooking, almost all the ingredients are easily available. Not only that, but these days you can find the complete dishes in restaurants. Many of them are even available canned and frozen ready-to-eat on supermarket and ethnic market shelves. In chapters 14 and 15 we'll have plenty of delicious recipes for high-calorie vegetarian dishes and even complete meals. But right now we'll show some more of the many examples of how meatless meals can put on just as much—or more—weight than their meat-containing counterparts.

One of the constant favorites in meatless cuisines are pancakes and waffles. For our purposes, if we think of these dishes basically as "carriers" of calories, we can put them to very good use. For example, 3 of the basic 4-inch-diameter pancakes made from a standard mix will give us about 350 calories. But that's before we start to enhance them. If we add only 2 tablespoons of oil to the batter, that brings up those piping hot little delicacies to a satisfying 600 calories. Then add butter and syrup for another 225 calories to get a grand total of 825 calories for 3 little pancakes.

But that's only the beginning. We can add toppings and include other appetizing items in the recipes to further fortify the caloric value. There are dozens of varieties of pancakes that we have never tasted and yet are favorites around the world. We can do the same thing for waffles with the same sensational results. You'll be surprised and delighted with the tasty recipe you'll find for pancakes in chapter 15.

There's an old standby that we can teach some sensational new tricks to help us put on pounds effortlessly. Pasta has always been high up on the menu for vegetarians, and there's a good reason for it. But now we can crank up the calories in pasta more than ever before possible. If you eat pasta made from white flour, you'll find you can consume plenty of calories without getting full or even feeling the calories as they go in. Take macaroni with cheese, for example. Just 8 ounces will give you 300 calories and if you put a little butter or olive oil on top of the cooked macaroni—say a tablespoonful—it comes out to 425 calories per serving. That's the equivalent—approximately—of a quarter pound of meat.

But let's see how we can turbocharge that pasta so it gives us even more calories in each bite. The new magic comes from a new invention—the motorized pasta machine. It's a home version of the commercial factory machines that has supplanted those charming but limited crank-driven chrome rollers. Now it's possible to get a fully automatic machine for less than $100 that will make our pasta automatically and exactly according to our specifications. And those specifications can be as high calorie as we want.

The machine is simplicity itself. You just mix the indicated amounts of flour, water, egg, and oil in a little see-through chamber. Then you press the button, and it mixes the dough. Hit another button and the pasta of your choice comes rolling out, extruded as if it were squeezed through a bunch of toothpaste tubes—which is pretty much what happens. The pasta is automatically forced through small (or large) holes. It passes over a warm drying current of air and drops onto a tray, ready to cook. You can make spaghetti, macaroni, ziti, manicotti, lasagne, and a whole slew of other kinds of pasta. You can also make cookies, pretzels, and a lot of other enhanced breadstuffs on the same machine in the same way.

But here's the wonderful advantage. You control the mixture. You can add just the amount of oil and eggs you want. The commercial pasta has little or no oil—because oil is one of the most expensive ingredients. In the same way, most commercial pasta has little or no egg, because eggs are very expensive. Whatever egg it may have is usually dried or commercial egg and in token amounts.

But you can actually make the best pasta in the world, because you can add the ingredients that Italian grandmothers used a century ago (and some still use today) to make pasta the way pasta should be made. Even more important, in the process, you will be making really high calorie pasta that will help you reach your weight-gain goal far faster than the store-bought commercial variety. Your best bet is to follow the instructions that come with the pasta machine.

Of course, if you don't have a pasta machine or don't want to get one or prefer not to make your own pasta you can still enhance your pasta dishes to get plenty of calories and get excellent results on your diet. It's just that occasionally new technology—like the pasta machine—comes along that can really help us in our program.

There's another machine that can really make a difference. It's the automatic bread machine. Selling for about $100, it's the equivalent of the automatic pasta machine but even a bit more versatile. You pop the ingredients—flour, liquid, salt, sugar, oil, and flavorings—into a chamber in the machine. Then you set a timer, push a button, and go away. You can even set it for 7:00 A.M. the next morning if you wish. The machine mixes the ingredients, drops in yeast if required, kneads the dough, lets the dough rise, bakes it, and then turns itself off when the bread is done!

Now, just think of the possibilities! There are also a lot of tasty ways to add calories by putting them on top of the bread. We can spread it with butter, peanut butter, jam, jelly, and lots of other things. But for the first time, the bread machine gives us a way to add calories by putting them inside the bread. We can add oil to the mix to crank up the calories. We can add extra eggs or sugar to do the same. We can add nuts and raisins and anything else to make the bread tastier and more caloric. If we get those extra calories inside our bread, we will hardly even notice them when we eat the bread, but they will be there working for us every step of the way. If we add calories to the inside of our bread at the same time we add them to the outside, gaining weight on a vegetarian routine will be even easier.

The nice thing about the bread machine is that it's practical for noncooks as well as experts in the kitchen. If you can tune in a channel on your TV, you can bake your own bread. Just pop in the ingredients, according to the easy recipes that come with the machine, set the time you want the bread to be ready, and hit the "On" button. You get superfresh high-calorie bread, ready just waiting for the addition of any one of a dozen enhanced toppings to put on pounds fast.

As if that were not enough, there is an extra plus. Everyone who has tried it knows that there is no substitute for fresh-from-the-oven bread. The physical-chemical process of subjecting the mixture of wheat flour and yeast to moist heat liberates certain flavor components that are impossible to duplicate in any laboratory or to add artificially.

In a certain way, hot bread fresh from the oven is like a kiss. You wait and wait for just the right moment. When it finally arrives, you can't hesitate. You have to seize the moment of pleasure—and suddenly it's over, before you know it! All that remains is the memory and the eager anticipation of the next opportunity.

But that's one of the important secrets of success of the vegetarian version of the Quick Weight-Gain Program. Everything we eat on that diet should be good—but really good! It should be lip-smacking good. As our Spanish friends say, it should *"traer agua a la boca"*—bring water to your mouth. That's because to gain weight on a vegetarian diet we have to overcome one little potential problem. The problem is simply this: vegetarian diets are basically "anorganoleptic."

That's a word that we medical doctors use and really it's a kind of shorthand to describe a whole series of events. (Honestly, we don't try to make up big words. Doctors don't really like big words but the scientific events that go on inside our bodies are often too complicated for little words.) "Anorganoleptic" means that vegetarian diets are usually "blah"—lacking in flavor and excitement. They are not organoleptic. And organoleptic is what a diet has to be to make you want to eat a lot of it.

Organoleptic comes from the word *organ* and the word *lepsis,* which means "seizure." So organoleptic is something that "seizes your organs." In the case of diet, it refers to a food that grabs hold of your sense organs—including smell and taste and touch—and won't let go of them. If your food isn't stimulating and exciting in a sensory way, you will find it boring and unattractive, and you will eat less. (Incidentally, that's one of the ways certain foods got their reputations as sexual stimulants—they stimulate the entire body and the sexual impulses at the same time. Some good examples are ginger and hot peppers in the Western cuisine and ginseng and others in the Oriental cuisine. We'll talk about some more of the sexual aspects later on.)

Here's a down-home example of an organoleptic food at work. Think of the last time you sampled freshly baked bread. As you cut off a slice of hot-from-the-oven (or bread-machine) bread, the aroma gets to your nose even before the bread gets to your lips. As the pungent yeasty fragrance saturates the scent receptors in your nose, you begin to salivate involuntarily. When the warm bread touches your mouth, you feel the heat and the consistency of the firm yet spongy bread. In the same few moments you have flavors and textures "seizing" the organs of taste, smell, and touch simultaneously. Of course you see the bread as you eat it, appreciating the contrast between the deep brown crust and the pale white bread. You can even hear the "crunch" of the crisp crust as you bite into it.

So in one single experience of eating, you experience the entire organoleptic phenomenon. Every one of the five senses is stimulated intensely and nearly simultaneously. That is precisely what we need to make eating as exciting and as pleasant as possible, so that we are constantly motivated to eat. Ideally we should look forward to eating, we should think about eating, we should anticipate eating. And we can only do that if eating is exciting.

That's one of the challenges in the vegetarian diet. Meat has the advantage of being eminently organoleptic. That steak sizzles in our ears, the rich meaty aroma races up our nostrils, we watch the juices swirl on the surface of the meat. The taste of the meat awakens our taste buds and the crisp and tender textures of the broiled steak press against our tongue as we eat it.

But how do we reproduce that intense, almost-simultaneous stimulation of every sense over and over again in our vegetarian diet? One way people have tried it is by adding "simulated" meat to their meals. These are ingenious and interesting products that are designed to look like meat and taste like meat, although they don't contain any meat at all. They come in many sizes and shapes—some are commercial and some are homemade. Many of the commercial products are based on a substance called "gluten." Gluten is a basic protein component of flour and the most common version is made from wheat flour. You can buy gluten at most health food stores, and in many supermarkets.

The gluten version of imitation meat is usually a brown and slightly spongy product that absorbs flavors readily. Another imitation meat is made from soybeans and has a variety of textures ranging from firm to spongy. The commercial products have the advantage of being easy to cook—just pop them out of their cans or boxes. And there are certainly plenty to choose from. There is no-chicken chicken, no-meat hot dogs, no-meat stew, and a myriad of others. With the right sauce and the right spices—and a little imagination—they come close to meat. Calories? That varies a lot depending on the product. Some are relatively high in calories, while others are only average compared to meat.

However, they fill a special niche. There are some vegetarians who don't like meat or anything that resembles it. There are others who don't eat meat for ethical reasons but still have a taste for something "meaty." These vegetable products fill the bill for them. You can find them in many variations at your local supermarket or health food store.

Homemade versions can be made from finely chopped mushrooms—the famous "mushroom-burger." But the most impressive "simulated meats" that exist are the Oriental versions. By a masterpiece of ingenuity going back centuries, they imitate duck, ham, and even barbecued spareribs. They aren't meat but they are certainly very close. (Recipes for these variations can be found in most Chinese vegetarian cookbooks.)

If it doesn't appeal to us, we don't have to use meat substitutes to make our weight-gain program attractive and exciting. But we can all benefit if we make our food much more organoleptic and exciting to all our five senses at mealtime—and in between times as well. One of the easiest ways to do that is by the judicious use of spices. Let's take one of the best-known regional diets—that of Mexico—as an example.

The traditional Mexican diet is basically a vegetarian diet. The basic foods are thin corn cakes called tortillas, mashed beans, and cheese. The peripheral foods are greens and vegetables like tomatoes, onions, etc. Another staple in the diet is, of course, rice. But corn, beans, and rice are bland and boring to the palate.

There is no excitement to the senses in eating a plate of rice or a dish of beans or a dry tortilla. So over the centuries the Mexicans have added powerful organoleptics to their basic diet. Their best-known—but far from the only organoleptic—is chili peppers. There is probably nothing in this world that stimulates all five senses as strongly as a nice hot chili pepper.

Hold one in your hand. It looks impressive—bright red. Raise it to your nose. It smells impressive as it makes your nostrils tingle. Bite into it and hear that distinctive crunch. A split second later you experience the texture and then—the unforgettable taste grabs you in its spectacular grip.

But that's not the way Mexicans have been eating hot peppers for centuries. They start very slowly when they are young. Just a tiny bit added to a big plate of rice or mixed in with the mashed beans. Then slowly and gradually over a period of years they increase the amount and the intensity of the peppers. And they know, as does every society, which peppers are the hottest and which are the mildest.

That's the secret. There are chili peppers so mild you can eat them like green peppers and only feel the tiniest bit of heat. There are others—usually small and harmless looking—that will set your entire digestive system ablaze for a week. It pays to know the difference.

Who can dare to eat those hottest of peppers? Here's the secret. Over time, most people develop a tolerance to hot peppers. The active ingredient in the pepper, "capsicum," gradually affects them less and less and they need larger and larger doses to get the same effect. (No, it's not addiction. It's "tolerance"—an entirely different phenomenon.) By the time they are adults, they can eat a hot pepper whole like a carrot or a cucumber.

But you shouldn't—unless your mother started you with a little tiny bit of chili pepper in your baby food. However, an infinitesimal amount of hot pepper in an otherwise bland dish will make your vegetarian weight-gain program that much more enjoyable, that much more efficient, and that much more successful. You'll find all the details, suggestions, and recipes in chapters 14 and 15.

You can get the same benefits in the vegetarian version of the Quick Weight-Gain Program taking advantage of other organ-stimulating ingredients like black pepper, vinegar, onions, garlic, and ginger. They will make your food more exciting and actually stimulate you to eat more at any particular time. When you utilize them selectively in your diet, you get a combination that excites the taste buds of people from cultures all around the world—and adds pounds at the same time.

With that in mind, let's take another look at that tortilla-beans-cheese combination. Now take the tortilla, mix some garlic and hot chili (a little or a lot) into the mashed beans, and spread the bean mixture on the tortilla. Sprinkle some chopped onions on top, add some grated cheese, then a splash or two of tomato sauce with various spices ("taco sauce," or as it is called in Spanish, "salsa de taco") and you have a mouthwatering, organ-stimulating dish.

Rice is another excellent example. Who likes rice? Well, some people may like rice pudding or something like that once in a while. But that's it. Let's face it. Rice, the way most Americans eat it, is about as "blah!" or "anorganoleptic" as anything can be. Strangely enough, almost everywhere else in the world, a plate of well-spiced rice can make anyone's mouth water.

Let's see a comparison of a standard rice dish and an organoleptic or sense-stimulating rice dish. Take the old standby, fried rice. Here's the standard U.S. version:

Rice, onion, 2 tablespoons oil, green pepper, canned mushrooms, egg, and soy sauce, all fried up together.

That's hardly something to make your senses leap to attention. Most Americans would probably end up putting ketchup on it.

Now, here's a vegetarian version of Thai fried rice. While it may not be just exactly to your taste, it's a good example of adding organ-excitement to a dish. A lot of people will like it just the way it is and we can always tone it down to suit our specific wishes. Here are the ingredients:

Rice, 6 tablespoons oil, minced garlic, chopped shallots, sliced ginger, tiny hot green chili peppers, bean sprouts, egg, and cilantro (Chinese parsley).

Now, that's much more inclined to sharpen your appetite than the standard U.S. version even if you cut down or eliminate the hot peppers. But that's not all. There's a sauce that goes along with the Thai fried rice that makes it even more stimulating.

It's made of ginger, a few more tiny hot peppers, more chopped shallots, and lemon juice. It also has a little bit of "red bean curd," a Chinese condiment made from soy that is similar to sharp cheese.

If we cook up this rice dish (or order it in a Thai restaurant), ladle on some sauce, and garnish it with fresh mint leaves, we'll know that we're eating something special. By the time we get all our senses working, we're not having a meal, we're having a total experience.

Most important of all, we will almost certainly find ourselves eating more than we intended. We'll put away twice as much rice and, in the process, 3 times as much oil. We'll get more calories and more pleasure—and we'll be more inclined to come back for the same dish a second time.

That, of course, is the whole idea of the Quick Weight-Gain Program. Each and every one of its concepts is aimed at encouraging us to eat more than we are eating now, both in food and calories, and to eat more often, so that we can easily and enjoyably gain the weight we so urgently need.

In the chapters that follow we are going to see exactly how to translate everything we have learned into a specific, detailed, day-to-day implementation of the most successful weight-gaining program ever designed: the Quick Weight-Gain Program.

## Chapter Eleven

# How to Help Your Child Put on Weight: "Menu Modules," Menu Modification, and Sebastian Q. Squirrel

I'm so worried! I'm about to go out of my mind! I've waited so long for this moment and now I'm about to lose everything!''

The woman who sat in front of me was well dressed, impeccably made up, and clearly well educated. She was also very very unhappy. She paused for a moment, then went on. "Doctor, I should mention that I don't usually lose control like this, but it's like the greatest crisis I've ever faced!''

"What seems to be the problem?''

"Let me begin at the beginning. Charles—that's my husband—and I have been married for eleven years. He's an architect and I'm an interior designer. That's how we met. Well, anyway we wanted desperately to have children and for some reason I just couldn't get pregnant. Finally, after years of treatment, little Andrew was born.''

She paused to brush a single stray strand of blonde hair away from her pale blue eyes. Those eyes suddenly reddened and filled with tears. "And now . . .'' Her voice broke.

"And now we're going to lose him!''

"Just a moment. What makes you so sure of that?''

"Oh, I just know it. He's so tiny and frail and he has that horrible disease that kills so many youngsters—you know, anorexia . . . anorexia . . .''

"Anorexia nervosa?''

"That's it! Poor little Andrew is so frail and so pale and he doesn't eat anything at all! Every day he gets thinner and thinner and there's nothing we can do to get him to eat!''

"How old is Andrew?"

"Hmmm. He'll be seven next month."

"How tall is he, and how much does he weigh?"

"He's about 3 feet, 11 inches tall, and he weighs about 51 pounds. But Doctor, he's just like a little toothpick! And we're going to lose him!''

"I don't think so. I don't think anything is going to happen to Andrew—except that pretty soon he's going to put on some weight. But let's take a look at him to be sure. Can you bring him with you next time?''

Suddenly she brightened. "I won't have to! He's in the waiting room with my husband! I'll get both of them!''

In a moment, all three of them were in my office. Andrew was a pale thin little boy with a look that managed to combine defiance with boredom. Charles was in his late forties, clipped mustache and clipped British accent. He spoke. "Caroline told me that Andrew has a chance to beat his disease. I'm delighted."

"Where did your wife get the idea that Andrew had anorexia nervosa?''

He frowned. "She saw a whole television program about it. You know, one of those afternoon panel-interview shows with 4 or 5 people with the same condition."

"Well, I have good news for you. Andrew is as likely to have anorexia nervosa as you are to have PMS. Anorexia nervosa is almost always a disease of young unmarried women. It's almost unknown in males and certainly not before the age of puberty. Let's get a complete physical exam of young Andrew and then we'll know more. But you can be sure he doesn't have any fatal disease.''

A week later they were in my office again. They were both obviously anxious and little Andy was as unperturbed as before. It was Caroline who spoke first. "I haven't been able to sleep for a week! Please tell us! What's Andrew's diagnosis?''

"This may come as a shock, but he doesn't have one. At least not a regular medical diagnosis. He doesn't have a metabolic problem, he doesn't have an absorption problem, he doesn't have a utilization problem. He—''

Charles interrupted. ''But then, Doctor, for the love of Heaven, what *does* he have?''

''Andrew has an eating problem. He doesn't eat enough.''

Charles looked at Caroline. ''By George, he's right! I've told you for years, that boy just doesn't eat!'' He turned to me. ''But now tell us, Doctor. What do we do with him?''

''You don't actually have to do anything with him. It's not that serious a problem. All we have to do is encourage him to eat.''

That's what we did, and within a month little Andrew was taller and heavier and much more cheerful.

An underweight child is often a source of chronic worry to his parents. In children weight is a symbol of good health as well as a gauge of growth. From the time a baby is born, parents assess his development more on the basis of his weight than anything else.

Of course, it is important for a growing child to constantly increase his weight. But almost invariably, underweight in a child before the age of puberty is the result of *how* they eat as much as *what* they eat.

Let's take a typical example. Children who are thin at the age of 5 or 6 usually have had eating problems long before. They were the ones who would spit out their baby food and push a plate off the high chair tray. By the time they are 5 or 6, they have developed a regular pattern. It goes something like this:

Mother serves lunch—let's say a cheese sandwich, some boiled potatoes, some peas, and a small mixed salad. Plus, of course, a glass of milk.

Junior looks at his plate as if it was overflowing with boiled worms. He listlessly takes a bite out of his sandwich, makes a face, and puts it down.

His mother frowns.

He picks up his fork, pokes at the peas, eats one, then spits it out.

Mother, annoyed, says, "Eat your lunch!"

Junior picks up a lettuce leaf, looks at it, takes a small bite and puts it down. He takes another bite of his sandwich, then starts to get up from the table.

"Where do you think you are going?"

"I'm not hungry! I don't want any more!"

And that's the end of another disastrous meal.

As every day goes by, Junior gets thinner, Mother gets more upset, and the problem becomes serious.

*Serious* is the right word because underweight in children is a more acute problem than underweight in adults. After all, adults have finished growing. Their basic organ and tissue structures are all formed and functioning. But with children it's a different story. Between the ages of 5 and 12 when most eating problems occur, children are in a critical stage of growth. That's when their little brains and nervous systems are developing, and it is well established that undernourished children tend to have lower intelligence levels than children with normal nutrition. But it goes far beyond that. Children who are underweight don't have nearly the same chance to develop in every way as children of normal weight.

There's another problem that is special for underweight children—they don't have that vitally important motivation to eat that is so essential if they are going to gain weight. A 27-year-old man who is underweight realizes that he has a problem and knows that he has to do something about it. A 7-year-old child only knows that he doesn't feel like eating.

What's the solution? Well, there are three techniques that can be combined to provide almost certain success in cases of childhood underweight. Each technique is simple in itself, but when they are combined, the results are almost always a pleasure to behold.

The first technique is "Menu Modification." Sometimes when we grow up we forget (perhaps because it was so long ago) that children have totally different tastes in food. If you offer smoked salmon, caviar, or Lobster Newburg to a 6-year-old, he is likely to screw up his face and in typical 6-year-old fashion say, ''Yuk! Don't you have any peanut butter?''

Children like special kinds of food. If you give them what they like, they will be much more inclined to eat. If you give them things they don't like, they won't want to eat them. But that's not really a surprise. That's exactly the way you and I feel, too. Think of it like this. In the Army or at camp or at a college dormitory cafeteria or an all-inclusive resort, even adults don't have much control over the menu. If they serve you something you don't like, you don't want to eat it. Well, in a sense, children are permanent nonpaying guests in an all-inclusive resort. They usually don't have any choice about what is being served to them. Their only defense is to not eat what they don't like.

But there's a problem. We've all been told over the years that children need a ''balanced diet'' to grow and develop. That balanced diet is supposed to consist of so many grams of protein, so many servings of green vegetables, yellow vegetables, eggs, and so many ounces of milk, etc. It's not supposed to contain sweets (rots your teeth!) or cookies or cakes or ''things that are bad for them.'' It's supposed to be full of ''things that are good for them.'' So the ideal diet for children is ''balanced'' and contains only ''good things.'' Sounds wonderful.

Now let's take the diet of an average adult. If you remove all the ''things that are bad for him or her'' from an adult's diet and replace them with ''things that are good for him or her'' and cut out the sweets and cookies and cakes, you'll see that he or she won't eat anything either!

Here's the real story. If you simply give a child what he wants to eat—and nothing else—he will get plenty of what he needs and he will grow and develop very nicely. There's plenty of proof of that. Take one interesting experiment done in a large orphanage. At mealtimes, instead of the usual rigid cafeteria system, they arranged all the possible food choices on a long table—buffet style. They put out cheese, cookies, fish dishes, desserts, fruit, vegetables, meat, chicken, and dozens of other dishes. They let the children, of various ages, walk down the table and pick whatever they wanted. Behind a screen the researchers wrote down what each child took.

The results were amazing. As you can imagine, the first day or so most of the kids took 3 desserts and a giant plate of pizza. No milk, no salad, no vegetables. But over the course of several weeks, they began to consume different foods each day. After a month went by, the researchers carefully compiled their lists and made an amazing discovery:

When their diets were carefully analyzed, each child was consuming a nearly perfectly balanced diet! Some days they ate a lot of starch, some days they ate very few vegetables. But when everything was added up, it came out to be a well-rounded and nutritious diet.

If we have an underweight child, it's hardly practical to set out a gigantic buffet at every meal time and let him choose from everything there. But we can make careful modifications in his menus that will encourage him to eat more and with less effort. With that in mind, let's take another look at that lunch:

Cheese sandwich
Boiled potatoes
Boiled peas
Small mixed salad
1 glass of milk

Now let's modify that lunch menu, according to the concept of "Menu Modification." Let's substitute what they call "fast food" for what is supposed to be "good food."

Here, in all its simplicity, is the modified menu:

Pizza with cheese and tomato sauce
1 malted milk

Sit your 6- to 10-year-old down to a lunch of pizza and a malted milk and you shouldn't have too much trouble. Did you ever notice a kid poking listlessly with his fork at a pizza? And the truth is that milk out of the cow doesn't have much taste. But if you make it into a malted milk, suddenly it becomes a flavor treat.

But how can this pizza-and-milk-shake lunch have enough nourishment? Well, let's look at the comparison. The cheese sandwich has protein and vitamin $B_{12}$, the bread has carbohydrate and vitamin $B_1$, the salad has vitamin C, and the milk has everything that milk has.

And the "fast-food" pizza? Let's see. It has protein and $B_{12}$ in the cheese. It has vitamin C in the tomato sauce—more vitamin C than the salad. The contribution of the potato and peas are insignificant especially since Junior doesn't eat them. The most nutritious food item in the world won't do you any good if you don't eat it!

Let's look more closely at the pizza. The pizza crust has everything that the bread has. As a matter of fact, a pizza is an open-face cheese sandwich with tomato sauce! Plus of course all the other nutritious things that you can put on a pizza like anchovies, sausage, green pepper, etc. You never thought of an anchovy as nutritious? Here are the figures:

A humble little anchovy is 19 grams of protein or about the same as porterhouse steak. It also contains plenty of calcium and phosphorus—essential for good bones.

The glass of milk is okay but the malted milk is superior in every way. The malted milk has more protein, more calcium, more phosphorus, much more iron, more vitamin A and more vitamin $B_1$, plus more riboflavin and niacin.

So the "fast-food" pizza and malted-milk lunch is a much better nutritional deal than the standard cheese sandwich meal. Most of us have been brought up to believe that "healthy" food has to be dull and tasteless food—as if eating is a chore that we have to do to keep ourselves alive. But that isn't true. If we make eating fun, especially for our children, they will eat and gain weight—and just as important, have a good time while they are doing it!

So if we want to add weight to underweight kids, give them what they want to eat and they'll get heavier, happier, and healthier. That's what Caroline did with Andrew. She tells it in her own words:

"I have to admit, Doctor, that I was shocked when you first outlined the Menu Modification idea for Andrew. But I was so fearful for his very survival that I decided to try anything."

"What happened?"

"Well, it was amazing. I started with lunch, as you suggested. I served him a hot dog on a bun with ketchup, pickle relish, and chopped onions. And then I gave him a nice big milk shake in a frosty glass. I'll never forget the expression on his face. It was a combination of delirious joy, total amazement, and the sneaking suspicion that his mother had gone stark raving mad."

"Did he say anything?"

Caroline laughed. "Yes, as a matter of fact he did. He said, 'Mom, who is this for?' And when I told him it was for him, he just started eating—stopping every few seconds to see if I was going to take it away from him!" Then she paused. "But I'm still wondering if I did the right thing!"

"Don't worry. Look at the nutritional facts. A typical 3-ounce hot dog gives you 12.5 grams of protein—that's more than half as much protein as a T-bone steak. It also gives you an abundance of calcium, phosphorus, iron, vitamin $B_1$, riboflavin, and niacin. The onions give you protein, calcium, phosphorus, iron, potassium, vitamin $B_1$, riboflavin, niacin, vitamin C, and vitamin A. The ketchup provides plenty of all the above vitamins and minerals plus a whopping dose of vitamin A. Even the pickle relish is high in calcium, phosphorus, and iron. And as for the—"

Caroline interrupted. "Excuse me, Doctor, but I see what you're doing! You're getting Andrew to do what he hates! You're sneaking a salad onto that hot dog bun!"

"Now you've got the idea! Of course. What difference does it make if he eats his salad from a nice hand-turned wooden salad bowl—or gets it on a bun with his hot dog? And he's getting the bread he doesn't want to eat on the hot dog bun. The milk shake gets him drinking the milk he despises—plus the extra calories he needs so badly.''

Caroline smiled again. ''I was just thinking. After all those years I spent at French cooking schools, I'm running a fast-food restaurant for my son—and I'm delighted that it's working!''

That's one tiny obstacle that sometimes stands in the way of getting children to eat. It's a kind of unintentional food snobbery that has been drilled into us. People sometimes say, ''You feed your children hot dogs?'' They usually say it as if a hot dog were some kind of pet food for hyenas. If we think about it for a moment, a hot dog is simply a ''wiener'' or a ''frankfurter,'' both referring to a food that originated in the noble cities of Frankfurt in Germany or Vienna in Austria. (In the Austrian language, *wiener* means someone or something that comes from Vienna.) These are the kinds of appetizing sausages that make up the daily diet of hundreds of millions of people. And if they make our children healthier and happier, so much the better.

Every parent knows what his child likes best to eat. To make Menu Modification as simple as possible, just give him those foods. And, for the moment, forget about the nutritional value—that will take care of itself. If you have any qualms, get a nutritional reference book at the nearest bookstore and look up the values of the so-called ''fast food'' that you are serving. You'll be pleasantly surprised. Pizza, hot dogs, hamburgers (another German city), peanut butter and jelly sandwiches, macaroni and cheese, barbecued ribs, and everything else that kids love—and don't see much of on the dinner table at home—are fine nutritionally.

Ethnic dishes are also especially popular with children and often they will eat them when they won't eat anything else. How often have you heard a parent complain, ''Little Roger won't eat a thing at home but when we take him to a Chinese restaurant, he eats everything in sight!''

Isn't that a clue? Why not serve him the same thing at home? But chop suey? How can a child grow and develop on something like chop suey? Aside from the fact that about a billion Chinese seem to have done very well on chop suey (or something very close to it), let's put the dish under our nutritional microscope and see what we find.

A typical plate of homemade chop suey gives you 10 grams of protein, or about what you'd get in cottage cheese. It also provides 48 milligrams of calcium, 200 milligrams of phosphorus, 4 milligrams of iron, 340 milligrams of potassium, 480 international units of vitamin A, .22 milligrams of vitamin $B_1$, .30 milligrams of riboflavin, 4 milligrams of niacin, and 26 milligrams of vitamin C. If your child likes chop suey, by all means give him chop suey.

Does your child like Italian fast food? Try a plate of spaghetti with meatballs in tomato sauce. Do you shudder at feeding a growing child an ''unbalanced'' meal like spaghetti with meatballs? Let's take a look at what it really offers:

A homemade plate of spaghetti with meatballs in tomato sauce will give your child a full complement of protein, vitamins, and minerals, including an abundance of calcium, phosphorus, iron, vitamin $B_1$, vitamin $B_{12}$, riboflavin, niacin, vitamin A, and vitamin C. How much of each of these essential elements will he get?

He'll get 7.5 grams of protein, 50 milligrams of calcium, 95 milligrams of phosphorus, 1.5 milligrams of iron, 268 milligrams of potassium, 640 international units of vitamin A, .10 milligrams of vitamin $B_1$, .12 milligrams of riboflavin, 1.6 milligrams of niacin, and 9 milligrams of vitamin C.

But is that enough protein, vitamins, and minerals? The answer to that one is easy. It's not a matter of ''enough'' nutrition. Whatever your child gets from the spaghetti with meatballs will be a million times more than he would get if he didn't eat at all.

Think of it this way. You can serve your underweight child a perfectly balanced high-fiber, organically grown, low-fat vegetarian lunch. If he is underweight, he will probably push the plate away, make a face, and that's it. Serve him a nice hamburger with all the trimmings on a crispy bun and he'll wolf it down. Which will do him more good? And remember that the hamburger (with the trimmings) is a well-balanced and nutritious meal.

But keep this in mind. Modifying your child's menu to feature fast food is only a temporary measure with one specific goal in mind—to help him gain the weight he so desperately needs to protect his health. Once his weight is back to normal, and you are sure it's going to stay there, you can gradually shift back to a more normal diet.

The truth is this: A perfectly balanced, high-fiber, organically grown, low-fat meal is ideal for a growing child. But if he won't eat it, he will get thinner and thinner and eventually suffer permanent damage from lack of nutrition. Once he's back to normal weight there's plenty of time to go back to a more traditional diet. But don't rush it—there's no hurry.

When you're doing "Menu Modification," there are some foods to avoid. For some reason (maybe metabolic), most kids have an aversion to foods that contain sulfur or strong flavors. That's why things like spinach and asparagus don't usually appeal to them very much. No matter what anyone tells you, these vegetables don't have any magic nutritional qualities. Don't force them on a child. As a matter of fact, it's not necessary to force any food on a child. Any food item that they don't like can always be substituted by something they do like of equal nutritional value.

Another thing to consider is the "fantasy foods" that crowd supermarket shelves. These are brightly colored, highly sweetened or highly salted bite-size morsels of something. They come in all kinds of shapes, sizes, colors, and flavors. They have bright exciting packages designed to attract small children but not much in the way of nutrition. These kinds of products are not helpful on a weight-gain diet.

"Menu Modification" means offering your child a range of foods to choose from that goes beyond the usual "meat and potatoes," but there has to be a limit and the limit is fantasy and entertainment foods. The guiding rule in "Menu Modification" should be, like in everything else, use your common sense. Be flexible, be inventive, be determined. But don't let Junior eat red-white-and-blue toasted jellybeans molded in the form of miniature Eiffel Towers in the hope that it will help him gain weight.

And remember, there is no magic in milk. The expression "Drink a quart of milk a day" was invented by a milkman, not a doctor. The only kind of milk that everyone should drink is mother's milk when they are a baby. Cow's milk is ideal for calves—you can drink it if you like it. But you can live your entire life healthy and happy without ever letting a drop of cow's milk pass your lips. If your children have eating problems, it isn't necessary to force them to "drink their milk," particularly since it is calves' milk, not *their* milk.

On that subject there's something else to consider. Sometimes children just don't like milk. Well-meaning parents may insist and nag and force the child to "drink his milk." They shouldn't. Milk isn't that important, and besides, the milk may be making the child sick.

Hundreds of millions of children in the world suffer from a hereditary condition known as "lactose intolerance." They are born without a particular enzyme called "lactase" that works to digest the lactose, or milk sugar, in milk. That means the undigested sugar just sits in the digestive system and ferments. That produces acid and gas and, often, diarrhea. Lactose intolerance is more frequent in children of African, Latin American, Oriental, and Middle Eastern origin, although it can affect almost anyone. Interestingly enough, children with that condition usually can tolerate yogurt and other fermented milk products easily, since the sugar has already been processed.

To help a child gain weight, the next step after "Menu Modification" is "Menu Modules." Underweight children often feel overwhelmed by an ordinary meal. They see too much food on their plate and they develop a kind of inner panic, because they're afraid they can't please their parents by finishing it all. Their infantile solution is not to eat anything! But if we break the food down into Menu Modules, we make life much easier for everyone. For example, if you are just starting in on a weight-gain program with a child, you can offer him pancakes for breakfast. But make them *little* pancakes for little mouths and little eyes. We really wouldn't like to sit down to a meal with a pancake the size of the Sunday paper, would we? Well, that's how big a normal adult pancake looks to a 6-year-old.

Make the pancakes about the diameter of a coffee mug so you could fill a mug with them if you had to. Then each one is just a bite or so for a kiddie, and they never feel threatened or overwhelmed. Do the same thing with sandwiches. A nice big grown-up sandwich almost makes a small child disappear behind it. Cut it into quarters or eighths—in triangles or other interesting shapes. And if the child doesn't like the crusts, cut them off and give them to the dog. The dog will love them and the child will learn to eat them someday—and if not, his health won't suffer seriously for lack of bread crusts.

That brings us to another point. When you feed your dog or cat, you just dump the food in the bowl and let the animal gobble it up. But if you are feeding a child, it pays to make the food look interesting and attractive—even artistic and cute. The more interesting food is, the more we want to eat it. A good example is Oriental cooking where the food is presented in fascinating shapes and interesting colors. The vegetables that are cut and peeled to look like flowers almost leap into our mouths. A fish that is decorated and adorned makes us eager to try it. That doesn't mean you have to take a course in Oriental cuisine to encourage your 7-year-old to eat. But if you go to a little extra trouble to make the food interesting and attractive, to get colorful dishes, napkins, and place mats, you may be pleasantly surprised with the results.

The final stage in solving a child's weight problem is the simplest and most effective. All you have to do is reward him for eating. Sound too easy? Let's think about it a moment. All our lives we have been told that eating is a ''duty'' and a ''privilege.'' Remember, ''Get to the table on time!'' ''Eat and be quiet!'' ''Get your elbows off the table!'' ''Chew with your mouth closed!'' ''Sit up straight or the food will go down crooked!'' ''Finish every morsel of food on your plate!'' and that wonderful non-sequitur: ''Think of all the poor children who don't have anything to eat!'' (It reminds me of the famous and very fat comedian who insisted that being fat was a sacrifice he willingly made. He used to say, ''See these rolls of fat that I carry around? I did that to save millions of children. My mother always used to say: 'Finish everything on your plate. Think of the children who don't have anything to eat!' And I did. And look at me now!'') Incidentally, by eating our food, aren't we actually taking food away from all those poor children?

Anyhow, eating should be fun, and one way to make it fun is to reward children who eat. Ron knows how it works.

"Jessica—that's my wife—and I really suffered with our daughter, Trudy. When she was 8 years old she only weighed about 47 pounds and she was really thin. She was short for her age and she just wasn't growing well. We tried everything you can imagine, except . . .''

Ron paused and looked serious.

"Except what, Ron?''

He looked at me and smiled. "We tried everything you can imagine, except the one thing that worked. We put that little girl through every kind of examination and every test and every treatment that anyone thought might work. We were really worried about her because she just wouldn't eat. Finally we got around to talking to you, and you suggested something so simple that I feel like a dummy for not thinking of it myself. And I'm supposed to be a brilliant computer programmer.''

"Don't blame yourself. Little girls are not computers.''

"Okay, but logic is logic no matter where you apply it. I remember you said, 'Make eating rewarding.' And that's what I tried to do. My wife prepared all the food in modules, like you suggested.''

"Give me an example, if you don't mind.''

"Glad to. For example, at dinnertime my wife served French-fried potatoes and little sausages—with plenty of ketchup and pickles on the side. Then she cut up little fingers of bread and spread them with peanut butter and jelly. Then she got out a big colorful place mat with a picture of a toy train on it. She found a plate with pictures of dogs and cats and a drinking mug like a clown. She served everything with all those pretty colors and it was really nice to look at. Especially, I guess, if you're 8 years old.''

''Then what?''

''Well, that's where I did my part, though actually any parent could do the same thing. The first time we made a special effort to set everything up very carefully in advance. We couldn't afford to fail. You see, Trudy, like most kids these days, loves video games and there's one game in particular with a little squirrel hunting for nuts in the woods that she's especially fond of. It's called ''Sir Sebastian Q. Squirrel and Friends.'' So I made this deal with her. For every 5 modules of food she ate, she got to play one game with Sir Sebastian Q. Squirrel. I was a little uneasy at first because it seemed too naive to expect it to work.''

''Did it?''

''Wow! You never saw food disappear off a plate so fast, Doctor! She just inhaled those French fries and sausages like she hadn't eaten in weeks. Then we went over to the computer and she played a game with Sir Sebastian. When it was over she raced back to the table, gobbled some more peanut butter and jelly fingers, and back to the computer. It was really hectic for a while—lunch table, computer, lunch table, computer. Finally I worked out a more relaxed system and we could sit through lunch.''

''What did you do?''

''Well, I printed out little tickets, so for every 5 modules she eats, she gets 1 ticket. And each ticket is good for a romp with her squirrel friend. She's been eating normally now for over a month, and Jessica is relaxed, I'm relaxed, and even little Trudy is obviously much happier. No more tension at mealtime, we sit through an entire meal without interruption, and best of all, she's gaining weight.''

You can adapt this system—really a very gentle form of behavior modification—to the needs of almost any child. Just pick an activity that the child enjoys and relate it to the consumption of various modules of food. The modules themselves are easy to make up. Just keep the individual servings small—about the size of a typical soda cracker is right, maybe a bit smaller for very young children. The module can be almost anything. Tiny pancakes are great, little squares of waffles and tiny sausages are excellent for breakfast. For lunch, if you are serving sandwiches, just cut each sandwich into small squares to make little miniature sandwiches. The idea is to make each module about bite-size—a nonthreatening, appetizing little morsel.

You can do the same thing with meat, pieces of cheese, pieces of pizza (our famous "camouflaged cheese sandwich"), carrot sticks, and almost any fruit or vegetable. Some things, like grapes and strawberries, already come in modular form. There is also an interesting psychological element in eating little portions of food. At cocktail parties and receptions you can observe that people tend to consume more food than normal because the hors d'oeuvres and canapés are tasty, tiny, and supremely easy to eat. If you think of a child's modular meal as a collection of hors d'oeuvres, everything falls into place. Just use your creativity and you'll be amazed at what you can come up with.

There are some aspects of behavior modification that apply particularly well to underweight children. The reward should be simple and immediate. That is, it's better not to promise a trip to the circus 3 weeks in the future. At first it's better to do what Ron did—the reward follows the eating immediately. Eat the 5 or 10 modules, and it's straight to the rewarding activity. That activity should be simple, not usually available, and something the child really likes. Playing a computer game, getting a colorful stamp to put in an album, getting another bright bead to put on a necklace. That's the kind of thing that's ideal for smaller children. For older children, they can earn pieces to complete a set. For example, with each set of modules they eat, they can earn a different piece required to build a model car. Or they can earn part of the outfit of a doll—if the components are small enough to be awarded just for consuming a set of modules.

That's the key to success at first. The reward should be simple, direct, and above all, immediate. Once a more stable eating pattern is established, the reward can be slightly more abstract, like the tickets that Ron printed. And the time period can be stretched—but not too much. For example, the reward can be later in the day—but in the early stages it's better not to extend it to the next day. As you go along you'll be able to adjust your child's responses and adjust the type of reward and the timing to get the best possible results.

There's one other thing you can do to help your child gain weight. It's so simple and so obvious that it's easy to overlook it. It's just this. Make sure your child has plenty of exercise every day of his life. There are few things more effective in building a healthy appetite than good physical exercise and in children it is a must. If you observe young animals—puppies and kittens, for example—you see that they are constantly running and frolicking, wrestling and rolling around. It's a natural and essential part of their development process. It's vital for your child as well. Get him to the playground, the school yard, the backyard, or somewhere where he can come back tired and hungry for lunch and for dinner. Keep him away from the TV and the computer and anything else that is sedentary. Any strenuous activity—swimming, running, dancing, jumping, playing ball—will do the trick. But make sure it happens. It won't solve the problem by itself, but it is the cheapest and easiest way to make sure that everything else you are doing will produce the desired results.

What about medicine for gaining weight? Some years ago it was fashionable to give children injections of hormones to increase their appetite and help them gain weight. Unfortunately some of these hormones were simply steroids or versions of male sex hormones. They could put weight on children all right, but they could also interfere with the growth of their bones and distort their normal sexual development. Don't even think about it.

The only medication you might consider is a simple multivitamin tablet. While there is no magic in vitamin pills, sometimes the vitamin $B_1$ or other vitamins in the pills do stimulate the child's appetite. They are worth trying, but only use the vitamins made specifically for children and only use the dose stated on the label.

Is it worth all that trouble? After all, why should you go through all the work of "Menu Modification," "Menu Modules," and behavior modification? The answer to that depends on how much you love your child. If you don't mind seeing him underweight and under par, if you don't care if he grows normally or not, then it's not worth the trouble. But if you want to give him the best you can—the best this world has to offer—it's worthwhile doing everything possible to help him achieve his normal weight—and a normal life.

## Chapter Twelve

# Seniors Can Do It Too: When More Pounds Mean Longer Life

**M**aybe my problem is that I'm too healthy!''

She chuckled as she said it. About 66 years old, dressed in a pale blue pantsuit with her abundant white hair held back with a jaunty red silk scarf, my patient seemed cheerful and unconcerned.

"What do you mean, Mrs. . . . ?''

"Call me Miss Lila—that's what all my students called me for the 35 years I spent teaching. I've been a high school teacher all my life—art and art appreciation—and I've always enjoyed studying. My husband was a hospital administrator—he died two years ago—and so I've had plenty of exposure to medical topics. I know what you doctors always say, 'The thinner the better,' and I've always tried to follow it. For years it was such a struggle. Would you believe that I once weighed 150 pounds?''

"That's interesting. How tall are you?''

"Five feet 5.'' She shook her head. "And now I only weigh 107 pounds.''

"Let's see. When you weighed 150 pounds you had a Body Mass Index of 25. That was decidedly overweight.''

"You bet!''

"But now at 107 pounds your BMI is a mere 17.88. And that's definitely underweight.''

She frowned and rolled up the sleeve of her blue jacket. "Don't I know it! Look at this arm!''

It was a thin, almost scrawny arm.

"But why have you lost 43 pounds?"

She smiled again. "If I wanted to be flippant, I'd answer something like: 'That's what I'm asking you, Doctor.' But it's more complicated than that. Actually I lost down to 125 pounds because I was just too fat. They used to call me Slim when I was in college, and I never wanted to be pudgy. But now when I hear the name, Slim, I want to cringe!"

"I can understand that. But tell me more. How is your appetite? Have you been sick lately? When did you see a doctor last? Let's get to the bottom of this!"

After an hour or so of thorough examination and probing, we discovered the following:

Miss Lila had maintained her weight at about 125 pounds until about 3 years ago, giving her a BMI of about 20.8—well within the normal range. But then, for no apparent reason, her weight began to fall off. Her appetite declined, and she just began to eat less.

"But why did you start to eat less?"

"I really don't know, Doctor. It was as if food suddenly lost its importance. For example, at lunch time, if I was busy drawing, I didn't feel like interrupting it just to eat."

"Just to eat" is a familiar phrase among people who are underweight, especially those who are older. Whenever you hear someone say that phrase, it brings to mind our old friend, the Opioid Feeding Drive. With advancing age many people lose that built-in urge, the emotional compulsion to eat, that drives billions of human beings to the meal table 3 times a day. When that inner compulsion to eat fades, their total food intake begins to fall off, and their weight declines. The Opioid Feeding Drive is comparable (although not identical) to the inborn pressure to breathe.[1] We breathe 18 or so times a minute without even thinking about it. Imagine how complicated life would be if we had to think about every breath! In a similar way, we gravitate to the dinner table (or restaurant or cafeteria or mess hall) 3 times a day, without even thinking about it. But many older people have to make a deliberate, conscious effort to prepare a meal, serve it, and eat it. For many, the incentive is lacking, and they are reluctant to make the effort "just to eat." That can lead to a lot of problems, including some that few people are even aware of.

For example, in the world of medicine there is an unusual disease condition that corresponds to the decline of the Opioid Feeding Drive. It particularly affects elderly widows living alone who gradually lose the Opioid Feeding Drive. With it goes their initiative to prepare and serve meals. So they settle for a cup of tea (or coffee) and a slice of toast day after day. A few months later they suffer a strange kind of weakness along with a gradual weight loss. When they finally consult their doctor, he finds an unusual kind of iron deficiency anemia from undernutrition that has come to be known in medical terms as the "Tea and Toast Syndrome."

The underlying problem is a serious one with older people because as they lose their interest in eating, they barely realize that they are missing meals and missing calories. But even though they may be sedentary, that calorie and a half is burning off their bodies as every minute goes by.

At the same time they lose the drive to eat, they are being cut off in the other direction. Remember when we looked into the effect of cholecystokinin on eating and appetite?[2] It turned out that when food leaves the stomach, it triggers the release of that substance, cholecystokinin. Its effect is to tell the brain that we are full—we couldn't eat another bite! It serves a very useful purpose if we are 25 years old and stuffing ourselves at the Fourth of July picnic. It can save us a lot of indigestion. But someone who is 66 years old and just barely maintaining his weight doesn't need anyone or anything to tell him he is so full he can't eat another mouthful. The problem is that older people often become overly sensitive to cholecystokinin secretion.

Even just a little bit—the amount that wouldn't affect a 25-year-old in the slightest—can shut off their appetite before they have barely begun to eat.

If that sounds like a lot of problems, don't worry! There is a solution to every problem, and gaining weight is what we are going to do. The first step in solving the problem of underweight in older people is to go right back to basics—a trip to the doctor for a thorough medical exam. Here is a summary of the 11 most important tests.

1. Complete blood count
2. Sedimentation rate
3. Urinalysis
4. Chemistry multiphasic panel (CMP)
5. Chest X-ray
6. AIDS test, if appropriate

There are 5 other special tests for special cases—your doctor won't overlook them, but you may want to remind him. They are:

1. Test for blood in stool
2. Sigmoidoscopy (flexible type)
3. Pap smear in women
4. Mammography in women
5. Prostate-specific antigen in men

Now, here's the good news! In almost half the cases of underweight, there is no evidence of serious physical disease. That's really encouraging when we consider that those are the years when cancer, heart attacks, strokes, and other degenerative diseases begin to take their toll. But then what does cause loss of appetite and weight loss in older folks?

As you can imagine, there are a lot of factors. As we medical doctors have done for years, the easiest way to look at it is to group the causes into major categories, 4 in this case. We can call it the "SPAM syndrome," for short. Here's the way it breaks down:

The first obstacle to normal weight in older people is *social*. So many of them are isolated and out of the mainstream of families. Too many of them live alone, where they are perfect targets for the "Tea and Toast Syndrome." They just don't have access to tasty food, well prepared and attractively served. And they don't have the emotional push to eat well and enjoy what they are eating.

The next obstacle is *psychiatric*. With advancing years all too many people suffer emotional declines. They are affected by depression, apathy, anxiety, and loss of memory. It's hard to do justice to a big meal if you are depressed and apathetic.

Another obstacle is *age*—pure and simple. As the years go by, many people gradually lose some of their sense of taste and smell. Unfortunately if you can't smell it, you can't taste it! (That's why little kids hold their noses when they have to take bad-tasting medicine.) Try the experiment yourself. The next time you are going to eat an apple, close your eyes and hold your nose. Ask yourself how many apples you would eat if they all tasted like that!

The final obstacle to good weight gain is *medical* problems. Even without any major diseases, older people often are missing teeth or have inadequate dentures, or arthritis that makes it hard for them to cook for themselves. In addition, many are taking various medications that can affect their appetite or upset their stomachs.

Then there are the serious physical diseases like cancer and heart attacks, diabetes, and strokes. These are things that have to be dealt with energetically by medical means and they are, of course, beyond the scope of this book.

But the other obstacles to weight gain are not really obstacles for us—they are challenges, challenges that we are eager and willing to overcome. Let's start at the beginning.

Eating is an eminently social activity. Human beings—and many animal species—have an inborn instinct to eat in groups. That's why we all sit down together to a meal. That's why we have restaurants and clubs, and family picnics and banquets and award dinners. Except for a small group of dedicated overeaters, people almost always eat significantly less when they eat alone. Without changing anything else, if we can get an older person to eat in a group—or at least with one other person—we will see their food intake increase. That's what we did with Miss Lila.

"Tell me, where do you usually eat your meals?"
She raised her eyebrows.
"Why, at the kitchen table, of course!"
"Do you eat with anyone else?"
"No, Doctor, I live alone, as you know."
"But you live in a senior citizens community, don't you?"
"Surely."
"But isn't there some kind of Community Center where you could get together for meals with other residents?"
She hesitated. "Yes . . . I guess there is. And some people do eat there, but it's so much trouble. I mean you have to haul all your food all the way over there."
"How far is it?"
"Oh, about a block and a half." Miss Lila smiled and shook her head. "I am being silly, don't you think? Of course I should eat with my neighbors instead of being holed up all alone in front of a TV in my tiny kitchen! I'll do it!"

That week, without doing anything else except starting to eat with other people, Miss Lila gained three-quarters of a pound.

Anyone who wants to gain weight—and that includes older folks, of course—should always look for the opportunity to eat in a group. If you are traveling and have to eat in a restaurant, look for someone else in the restaurant who is eating alone and see if you can join them. It doesn't take much—just say something like, "I notice that you are eating alone—would you like some company?"

Take advantage of every chance to eat with a group. Perhaps your church or social club has a program where people get together at mealtime. If they don't, you might consider organizing a program like that yourself. Remember the group doesn't have to be gigantic to be effective. Even eating with one other person instead of alone can make a difference. For example, if you notice that one of your neighbors seems to be eating solo, just tap on the door and ask if he or she would care to join you. You just might get a very pleasant surprise. If you eat with someone else, not only will you meet new and interesting people, but you will find it easier to eat more and keep to your weight-gaining goal.

The next obstacle we have to overcome is the psychiatric. That's really a medical problem, but not an impossible one by any means. Your doctor can often help with antidepressive medication or perhaps hormone replacement therapy in women suffering from hormone-deficiency depression. But whatever the cause, psychiatric conditions that depress appetite have to be brought under control before we can really make substantial progress in gaining weight.

The specific problems caused by the dulling of the senses of taste and smell with the passage of the years aren't really obstacles if we know how to attack them. So many older people make the mistake—because of what they have been told over the years—of eating bland and dull foods. They are afraid of "upsetting their stomachs" or "getting indigestion." So they eliminate spices and condiments and strong-tasting and strong-smelling foods from their diet. Then they complain that they don't feel like eating because their food doesn't have any taste! Of course it doesn't have any taste if they have taken all the taste out of it!

That's what Miss Lila and I discussed one afternoon.

"You know, Doctor, I never thought about it before, but when I grew up, food was a moral issue."

"A moral issue? What does food have to do with morality?"

"That's the point. Not much, but that's not the way I was brought up. According to my parents, you were supposed to eat just because you were supposed to eat. You took your food the way you found it. Putting spices or sauces on your food was considered—

well, kind of too fancy, too sophisticated, almost kinky. Like wearing your skirt too short.'' She giggled nervously. ''Don't ask me why! But that's the way they made us feel. And now when I start to put even Worcestershire sauce on a piece of chicken, somehow I feel guilty. I know it doesn't make any sense . . .''

Not only doesn't it make any sense, but those notions implanted in childhood can stand in the way of meaningful weight gain. Miss Lila was right—early attitudes toward food die hard. How many times have we seen a mother complain when a teenager sloshes ketchup all over his French fries? How many wives complain when their husbands drench a piece of meat with steak sauce?

You know the words: ''After all the trouble I went to, just to cook that meat for you! Look what you're doing to it!''

But there's something we should remember. The primary purpose of cooking is to feed the ones who are eating. If they enjoy steak sauce or even pink mayonnaise on their meat, it doesn't matter—as long as they enjoy it and benefit from it. It's the ultimate consumer of the food, the one who eats it, who is entitled to make the final decision.

Miss Lila was right about something else, too. For all too many people, there is supposed to be something vaguely immoral or ''just not right'' about food that is ''too fancy.'' Most of the time that doesn't matter—it's a question of individual taste and perception. But when we are fighting the battle of underweight in older people, we need every weapon we can get our hands on.

That means that any food that will stimulate appetites, encourage eating, and put on pounds is the right food for us. And any spice, sauce, or condiment that will make our food more attractive is right for us. But that goes double (or triple!) for older folks. They need more excitement in their food than before. (They also need more excitement in their lives, but that's another book.) They need spices and sauces and condiments that will brighten up the color, intensify the smell, and heighten the taste of what they are eating. They need all the help they can get so that the pungency and the power of the food can break through to their diminished taste buds and decreased sense of smell.

The first place to start is the supermarket shelves. Try, one by one, all the various sauces and salad dressings that you even think might appeal to you. And then try a few that you don't have any idea about—you just might be pleasantly surprised! The list can include all the many variations on barbecue sauce, including smoke flavor, chili, garlic, mushroom flavor, and anything else that strikes your fancy. After all, this is an eating adventure—you are prospecting for new flavors and experiences. Then try the full range of spaghetti sauces—with meat, with mushrooms, with cheese, and all the rest. Then you can hunt through the various types of ketchup—and there are more variations coming out every day. Then move on to mustards—there is the common yellow, the German brown, the French Dijon, and the horseradish-mustard combinations. Be adventurous and remember that it's all for a good cause—adding pounds. Don't forget the various forms of Worcestershire sauce and all the different steak sauces, and anything else that appeals to you.

Then check out the salad dressings. Remember that most salad dressings—except for the lo-cal that we don't even look at—have a lot of oil and therefore a lot of calories. Try every kind that even remotely seems interesting to you and you will surely find pleasant surprises. Try the Blue Cheese, Caesar, Cheese with Garlic, French, Green Goddess, Italian, Hawaiian, Russian, Tahitian, Smoky Bacon, Sour Cream, Thousand Island, and anything else that seems even the slightest bit appealing. The idea is to make eating an adventure—to make eating exciting again!

The next step is to try different cuisines. American and Northern European cooking is strong on basics—meat and potatoes. But Southern European, including Spain, France, Italy, Greece, and all the rest, emphasize exactly what older people need the most—strong flavors and strong aromas. Latin American cooking—especially Mexican—also puts the accent on flavors and aromas. But there is no cuisine like the Oriental for stimulating the taste buds and the sense of smell.

This was Miss Lila's experience:

"Well, I did what you suggested, Doctor, but it wasn't easy."

"Wasn't easy? Why not?"

"Well, you know, in this country we're not used to taking our eating that seriously and when you told me to go into a Chinese restaurant and talk to the cook! Well, I declare! I was really surprised!"

"But doesn't it make sense? You're paying for the meal and you have a right to ask for what you want. And in your case, you're not just ordering food, you're ordering medicine to save your life."

"Well, when you look at it that way, it makes sense. Anyhow, I picked the best-looking Chinese restaurant I could find and I found the manager. I was surprised that he was such a nice man and when I explained my problem he took me into the kitchen personally to talk to the cook. He told him a lot of stuff in Chinese and the only word I could make out was something like, 'Etch-One.' I didn't think they were going to draw my dinner but I was ready for anything. There was a lot of smiling and nodding and then the manager took me back in and sat me down."

"And then what happened?"

"I had to wait about 15 minutes and then they served me the best meal I ever had in my life! The amazing thing was that everything had a taste! It was spicy—but not too much. And it smelled almost like perfume! I ate so much that I could hardly get up from the table! Now I go there at least once a week and I march straight into the kitchen to see what new ideas the cook has come up with."

She paused. "And by the way, I found out what 'Etch-One' means. It really means, 'Szechuan,' the southern province of China where the food is supposed to be the spiciest and most exciting. And it certainly lives up to its reputation!"

Now, don't waste your time talking to the cook at your local fast-food emporium. He cooks according to a formula and it's always exactly the same. Beware of a new kind of restaurant—the ethnic fast-food restaurant. These are places that offer Chinese, Italian, Middle Eastern, and other ethnic foods made according to the same kind of uniform recipes that the everyday hamburger and pizza places use. There's nothing wrong with these establishments for ordinary eating—or even weight gaining under some circumstances. But for older folks who need to gain weight, the exciting smells and flavors of the home-style restaurants are more effective.

The best part of almost any home-cooking ethnic restaurant—Chinese, Korean, Japanese, Thai, Vietnamese, etc.—is that they usually will be delighted to discuss and explain the food to you. And they will help you choose the dishes that are the most pungent and most aromatic—the ones that will stimulate your appetite the most. Be adventurous. Be bold. Look for new experiences.

Of course, we have to be practical as well. Not everyone can eat all their meals at various ethnic restaurants. It's a matter of convenience and cost, among other things. There's something else to think about, too. Don't be tempted by the frozen dinners of ethnic origin. A frozen Chinese chow mein dinner or a Mexican beef enchilada dinner is fine for the average weight gainer. But if it's for an older person with an impaired appetite and a diminished sense of taste and smell, it's better to stick to the freshly cooked version. Freezing, defrosting, and reheating take too much of the sensory punch out of the ingredients.

But there's an easy solution for all that. In chapters 14 and 15, you'll find some recipes specially selected just for older people who need stronger flavors and stronger aromas to stimulate their senses and their appetites. It includes recipes from Mexico, Korea, China, Japan, Vietnam, and many other countries—specially chosen for their attractive appearance and appealing flavors. You can make them all at home quickly and easily—and the ingredients are easy to find. Actually most of them are on your supermarket shelves these days. You'll gain weight, you'll save money, and you'll have fun in the process.

Even if you don't feel especially like cooking from scratch, there are some very useful tricks you can use to make your menu more stimulating and exciting. The next time you go shopping, pick up a nice selection of spices from the supermarket spice rack. Be sure to include things like powdered coriander, powdered cumin, powdered garlic, powdered onion, curry powder, oregano, black pepper, dill seed, red pepper flakes (if you're the adventurous type), and anything else that even remotely seems interesting to you.

Then, when you sit down to eat—whether it's food from a can or a frozen dinner or even freshly made—just sprinkle a little of your favorite spice on your dinner. You'll improve the aroma, spark up the taste, and improve your appetite at the same time. Some of my patients even carry a few spices with them in their pocket or purse when they eat out. That's how they transform a so-so restaurant meal into something really tasty and attractive. Adding your own spices to processed or restaurant or institutional food can make a world of difference. You'll eat more and enjoy it more.

Sometimes, especially in older people, a little detective work comes in handy. Jim was a good example. At 68 he still had the military bearing that fitted with his career as a naval officer. A retired navy captain, he ran a small orchid nursery. He sat upright in his chair as he spoke.

"I just don't understand it. I eat well. As a matter of fact, I eat a lot. And I still don't gain weight! Actually, I seem to be losing!"

"How much do you weigh, Captain?"

He grinned. "Just make it 'Jim,' Doctor. All that's behind me. I weigh 137 pounds, and I'm 6 foot 1."

"Let's see. That gives you a BMI of 18.15—certainly underweight. But you say you eat a lot?"

Whenever a patient is losing weight, or failing to gain, in spite of a substantial food intake, we always worry about some very serious underlying disease. Cancer or leukemia are the ones that come to mind first. Two weeks later I was even more concerned about Captain Jim—especially since the tests that I had ordered all came back normal. But now I had different suspicions.

"Jim, can you tell me what you had for breakfast this morning?"

"Let's see. The usual breakfast. A couple of eggs, some toast, a little bacon. A few pancakes. Then some coffee."

"How about dinner last night?"

He hesitated. "Ummm. Last night? Yeah. A steak—medium rare—smothered in onions, a baked potato, some peas. Then a couple of rolls and butter . . . and uh . . ."

"Dessert?"

"Yeah, dessert. That was apple pie, I think. Yeah, apple pie."

"Jim."

"Yes, Doctor? What is it?"

"You don't really remember what you had for dinner, do you? Be honest."

"Uhmmm. To tell you the truth, I have so many things on my mind that I can't keep track of all that little stuff."

I spoke gently. "And the truth is, you really can't remember what you had for breakfast either. Isn't that right?"

Jim shrugged. "I suppose so. For the past year or so, I've been having to write everything down. I guess I should write down what I eat too—if you're going to ask me!"

"It wouldn't be a bad idea for a while—just so we can find out what's going on."

Sometimes older people have unreliable memories. It doesn't mean they have Alzheimer's syndrome—it's just something that can happen. Under ordinary circumstances, it's merely a nuisance, but if it makes them forget to eat or forget what they have eaten, it can cause problems. In Jim's case, he wrote everything down for a week and here was a typical example:

## BREAKFAST

1 slice of bread with jelly
1 soft boiled egg
1 cup coffee with cream and sugar

## LUNCH

1 tongue sandwich with mustard
1 can of beer
4 fig bar cookies

## SUPPER

1 frozen dinner—chicken with vegetables
1 can of beer

No pancakes for breakfast, no steak, medium rare, smothered in onions, no baked potato. It was all what we call in medicine "confabulation," or making up details of something you can't remember to try and conceal your lack of memory. "Confabulation" is more common in older folks than most people realize.

The solution in Captain Jim's case—and one that is ideal for everyone in his situation, if at all possible—was this. He moved in with his married daughter and ate all his meals with her, her husband, and their two children. He dropped in to see me two months later.

"How's everything, Jim?"

He chuckled. "Fine, Doctor. I've put back 9 pounds so far! But please don't ask me what I ate for dinner last night. They fill my plate, I clean it off, and no one asks any questions!"

It worked out fine for Captain Jim, and it can work for everyone.

There's another important element in overcoming underweight that's worth mentioning. Remember the tradition among the British explorers in remote areas of Africa and Asia in the last century? No matter how isolated or primitive their conditions were, they always dressed for dinner. It could be a small clearing in the jungle or a desolate site at the edge of a volcano—it didn't matter. They washed, shaved, dressed, and sat down to a nice meal.

Older people in particular need an attractive and appealing setting for eating. All the silverware dumped in a can, a knife stuck in a loaf of bread, and a greasy plastic tablecloth will not improve their appetite. They need, and deserve, an attractive table setting with a clean table, colorful place mats, matching silverware (stainless steel is fine), and a quiet, charming place to eat. A flower or two on the table, a bit of soft music on the radio, perhaps a candle in the evening will go a long way to enhance their food intake. Remember that's the way that restaurants do it. Why? Because they have found over the years that people eat much more when the setting is appealing. Of course, the more the customer eats, the more money the owner makes. At home, the more an older person eats, the more weight he gains—and that's what we're working for.

Another interesting hint from the restaurant professionals is this one. If at all possible, eat outdoors. Restaurants that serve food in patios or gardens have discovered that consumption increases significantly when the customers are in the fresh air. Try it at home—it doesn't take much. A few square feet under the sky is enough. For apartment dwellers, a spot by the pool (if your apartment has one) is fine. Otherwise an occasional trip to the park with a picnic lunch will help the cause of weight gain.

That brings us to exercise. More than any other specific measure, exercise can help older people to gain weight. It really does a lot of good things all at the same time. There's no question that regular exercise helps keep them in shape but more important, it also increases their appetite. At the same time, it produces a feeling of well-being that makes them more interested in life and concerned with putting back that lost weight.

The specific kind of exercise isn't too important, just so long as it's intelligent and appropriate. Mountain climbing wouldn't be right for most older folks, although it could be great for some individuals.

Walking around the block might be too little for the majority, although it could be perfect for someone who is especially old and delicate. The secret is to do what seems best for you. The ideal exercise is the one that produces a feeling of satisfaction, as if you've accomplished something worthwhile in the process. Walking, swimming, and noncompetitive, low-stress sports are ideal. The emphasis is on "noncompetitive" and "low stress." For example, tennis is fine and so is golf, provided they don't lead to increased tension and anxiety that interfere with your appetite and end up producing a further weight loss rather than a weight gain. Positive, productive exercise is our goal. Some of my personal favorites are yoga and Tai Chi Chuan—but everyone has to find the activity that's just right for them.

There's something else that older people can do to help themselves. In books on losing weight a lot has been written about allowing your stomach to shrink. The thought is that if you cut down on the bulk of food you eat, your stomach will get smaller. Then, hopefully, a smaller amount of food will begin to stretch it and you will feel full much sooner than you might if your stomach were regular size or bigger. The truth is, it's really hard to tell. The stomach is an elastic organ that can stretch and shrink pretty much as our food intake changes.

On the other hand, since no one really knows for sure, it just might be a good idea to try and stretch your stomach a bit so that you can eat more before you feel just too full. It could well be that in addition to cholecystokinin and the Opioid Feeding Drive, the physical capacity of our stomachs might influence our feelings of fullness. How to do it? The easiest—and most beneficial way—is just to eat a little bit more when you feel full. Just take another two bites after you think you've had enough. Gradually, almost imperceptibly, you will stretch your stomach (if it can really be stretched). And if you can't really stretch your stomach, you will be getting that many extra calories working for you. So either way, you win! And that's the way we like it!

Something else that will help older folks is protein. Most people get plenty of protein in their diet. Meat, eggs, fish, chicken, and all the milk products are loaded with protein. But older people have a higher rate of ''catabolism'' than younger people. Remember that in everyone new tissues are being created all the time while old tissues are being destroyed. The creation of tissues is called anabolism, and the destruction of tissues is called catabolism. When a child is growing, anabolism outpaces catabolism and the child increases in size and weight. During adulthood, anabolism and catabolism are pretty much evenly balanced, and size, if not weight, remains stable. But as the years go by, more tissues are broken down than are replaced and older people begin to suffer from atrophy of their tissues. Their muscles become flabby, their tissues become loose, and they gradually lose important structures. One of the things that helps them resist the breakdown that catabolism causes is a diet with adequate amounts of protein. The key words are ''adequate amounts of protein.'' Too little protein means they can't keep up with the tissue loss but too much protein puts an unnecessary strain on their kidneys, which ultimately have to deal with the protein load of the body.

There are all kinds of protein in this world but the one thing they have in common is that they are composed of amino acids. A protein is really like a necklace of pearls, and each ''pearl'' is an amino acid. There are about 22 of these amino acids in nature. Human beings can synthesize—produce in their own bodies—about 14 of these. But there are about 8 that we can't make on our own and we have to get from our food.* These are called ''essential amino acids'' and they include the following: tryptophan, leucine, lysine, methionine, phenylalanine, isoleucine, valine, and threonine.

The story of essential amino acids is really fascinating. For a protein to be truly useful, it has to have all the essential amino acids present. But that's not enough. They have to be there in adequate amounts for the body to use them to make more protein. For example, if a particular food has 100 percent of 7 of the essential amino acids but only 50 percent of the eighth, then it has only 50 percent

* We say ''about 22'' and ''about 8'' because in medical science, research never stops, and we are always making new discoveries.

of the value for making more protein. In a sense, the amino acid chain is only as strong as its weakest link. That's why older people should concentrate on getting their protein from the best possible sources—foods that contain all 8 of the essential amino acids in generous amounts.

The best insurance is to eat at least one good serving of meat or fish or chicken a day. A bit of cheese—cottage cheese is fine—will also provide extra insurance against protein deficit. But the thing to avoid is the "Tea and Toast Syndrome"—and it can come in many forms. Some older folks eat breakfast cereal for breakfast. Provided that it is enhanced, that's fine. But then they go on to eat it for lunch! And some even eat it three times a day. That exposes them to a low-protein diet with inadequate essential amino acids. Other times older folks eat a lot of sweets (like cookies) and starches (like potato chips and other salted snacks). They may feel full but they are almost always lacking in the essential amino acids.

What about vegetarians? Does an older vegetarian have to start eating meat just to keep healthy? Hardly. There are plenty of non-meat sources of essential amino acids including milk products like cheese, yogurt, and milk itself. They can also eat eggs, which have more protein and better quality protein than anything else, including beefsteak. There is another solution which most vegetarians know already. That consists of combining what are called "complementary proteins." If one food has a lot of most of the essential amino acids but is really deficient in one or two, why not eat it at the same time as you eat another food which has plenty of the missing essential amino acids? By a fascinating fact of nutrition, that's exactly what human beings have been doing instinctively for about ten thousand years.

Taken separately, rice and beans are lacking in some essential amino acids. But if you combine them, you get a dish that has as much of the essential amino acids as porterhouse steak! Almost everyone in Latin America from the richest to the poorest eats rice and beans in some form or another. The same holds true for beans and corn. So if you eat mashed beans (remember our "frijoles refritos''?) on corn tortillas, you might as well be eating sirloin steak as far as your protein is concerned. Another excellent high-protein combination is soybeans and rice—and soybean products are almost always combined with rice in Oriental cuisines. A cheese sandwich on whole wheat bread will also do the trick—and it's not a coincidence that a slab of cheese on whole wheat ''pita'' bread has been a staple for millions of people all over the Middle East for 50 centuries.

So, with a little scientific knowledge, a little common sense, and a lot of determination, together we can solve any problem that stands between us and the normal weight we need to achieve.

## Chapter Thirteen

# Making the Most of Your Diet: The Total Push for Pounds

**W**ell, I'm all set to go! I think I understand everything you've said. I have all the basic principles of weight gain very clearly in mind. But I just have one problem . . .''

Jennifer spoke those words. She was 31 and the mother of two children. She was the director of public relations for a large recording company and she was as dynamic and agitated as one of their hit records. She went on: "I have it all clearly in mind but the only thing I don't know is . . . is . . ."

I interrupted gently. "Is how to start?"

Suddenly she sat up straight in her chair. "That's right, Doctor! When do I start? How do I start? What do I do first?"

"The answers, in order, are *with your next meal, by consuming more calories,* and *plan carefully.*"

"Hmmm, that makes sense. Let's see how my schedule looks." Jennifer glanced at her watch. "Okay, it's 10:45. My next meal is at noon. I'm almost always in a hurry at lunchtime, so I grab a sandwich and a can of pop—usually at my desk." She looked at me sheepishly. "But I try to make it up by snacking in the afternoon."

She paused. "I know, I know. Those relentless one and a half calories a minute. There's no way to make up for them."

"You're right, Jennifer. If you're going to be successful in your weight-gaining program, you have to approach it like a military campaign. Your enemy is underweight—time is on his side—and what you don't take from him, he will take from you. Your first battle begins in an hour and a half; prepare yourself for it by planning your tactics carefully. Think it through.''

Jennifer frowned. ''Okay, but this is the first time I'm really getting serious about this problem. Can you give me some hints?''

''Sure, Jennifer. Do you have to eat at your desk?''

''To tell you the truth, most of the time, no. I've just gotten into the habit. Maybe that's why I weigh 99 pounds. But today I do have to stay at my desk to go through a presentation that I have to make at 1:30 this afternoon.''

''Could you have prepared for the presentation last night?''

A flush of bright pink rose from her neck to her forehead. She shrugged her shoulders. ''Sure, I could have. But since I never eat much lunch, I figured I could do it then . . .'' She raised her hand to her cheek in amazement. ''Uhhh! Now I see what you mean! Planning! Of course! If I'd been up-to-date in my work I would have had time for a relaxed lunch. But I've always considered eating to be the least important thing that I do.'' Her expression became serious. ''And that's probably why I weigh 99 pounds! Okay, what do I do today?''

''Is the presentation important?''

''You bet!''

''How does this sound to you? Order a nice high-calorie meal delivered to your office. Make a deal with yourself not to even glance at your presentation until you finish every single bite of your lunch. The idea is to give yourself an incentive to eat and convince yourself that you are changing the priorities in your life. Your health and your appearance and your very survival come before anything else.''

Jennifer smiled a knowing smile. ''If I didn't know any better, I'd think you were trying that behavior modification you use on children with me. You know, eat your hamburger and you get to play a video game. But you wouldn't do a thing like that, Doctor, would you?''

Now it was my turn to smile. ''If it could help a patient gain weight, I just might!''

Jennifer nodded. ''I thought so.''

''You see, the idea is this. Adults don't always need the same positive reinforcers as children. By the time we grow up, most of us are used to pursuing longer-term goals. In other words, we understand the psychological concept known as the 'Pleasure Principle.' We are used to giving up immediate satisfaction for future benefits.''

For most people food and eating qualify as ''immediate satisfaction.'' But for folks who are underweight, just eating isn't that exciting. On the other hand, we all have our responsibilities which we have to fulfill. So if Jennifer decides that she won't let herself prepare for an important meeting until she eats every bite of her high-calorie lunch, she suddenly gets all the benefits of behavior modification. Let's see if it worked.

I asked her about it on her next visit.

''How did that idea work out with lunch at your desk and the presentation you had to give?''

Jennifer laughed. ''It was almost too good, Doctor. I put the lunch on one end of my desk and the report at the other end and lined up the food in a row between me and the report. Then I told myself I had to 'eat my way' to the report. I was getting worried by then because I had only 35 minutes left.

''Well! I went through that meal like a termite through a woodpile! I had two hot dogs, an order of French fries, a big milk shake, and a piece of apple pie. And when I finished, I found myself looking around for more. Now I eat lunch at my desk two or three times a week because I've started to enjoy it that way. I put my work for the afternoon at the far end of the desk and make myself 'eat my way' to it. I've gained 5 pounds in the past two weeks and really had a lot of fun doing it!''

It worked for Jennifer, and it might work just as well for you. This is a ''negative incentive''—if you don't finish your high-calorie meal, you won't allow yourself to do all the other things you so urgently need to do. It works, but it requires a little help on your part. The key to success in behavior modification resides in two important words: planning and discipline.

The planning part works this way. Before each meal select a target task that absolutely has to be done within the next few hours—or at most, the next day. It can be making a telephone call to your lawyer, buying a birthday gift for your wife, finishing a project for your boss—anything that is vital to your happiness and success. Then plan a meal loaded with calories. It can be from any of the menus listed in chapters 14 and 15 or a selection of your own choosing. But it has to be really high calorie to count.

That's the first part. The other half of the technique is the discipline. Once you choose the target task and the meal, stick with it as if your very life depended on it, because *it does*. Remember that the sole purpose of behavior modification is to help you gain the weight you need to protect your health and avoid a premature and tragic death. When you select your task—whatever it is—resolve not to perform it unless and until you finish every bit of your meal.

Behavior modification is taking a hard line toward underweight. It works, and it justifies the discipline it takes. But there is another strategy that you can use to great advantage that uses an entirely different approach. And this one is fun—pure, unadulterated fun.

Brett tried it and it helped him immensely.

"Can you believe, Doctor, that I had gotten to the point where I actually dreaded mealtime? I knew I had to eat but all I wanted to do was get it over with as soon as possible. Back then—it was two months ago—I weighed 115 pounds and I'm 5 feet 7 inches tall. That gave me a BMI—you showed me how to calculate it—of 18. I was playing with fire, as you can see. I'm 39 years old and I'm an advertising account executive. It's the world's worst job for a skinny person. On the one hand I have to have a good appearance and on the other hand the job is overflowing with stress and tension. The greater the tension, the less I eat. And the less I eat, the worse I can handle the tension. That doesn't leave me with a lot of energy to take on more hard tasks. So when you suggested that there was an easier way to gain weight, I jumped at it.''

"I'm delighted to hear that."

"It all started when you told me how they used to treat mental patients—before the days of tranquilizers. I know I'm not a mental patient but being overworked and underweight at the same time really makes you tremendously tense and nervous. What attracted me was what you called the 'Total Push' technique. Do you remember?''

"Of course. Back in the days when there wasn't really much of a treatment for mental illness, some doctors came up with a new idea. They decided that if they couldn't do something specific for the patient, at least they would do everything they could to encourage him to heal himself. They remodeled the old somber mental hospitals and made them bright and cheerful. They planted pretty gardens with flowers and trees and they constantly played happy music for the patients. In effect, they did everything possible to offer a cheerful and positive environment to encourage the patients to progress on their own.''

"And that's what you suggested for me."

"Right. The whole idea was to make eating a pleasant experience that you would look forward to. Something that gave you satisfaction above and beyond the simple act of eating itself.''

"Boy, it sure worked! And it was fun doing it! Of course, a big part of the credit belongs to my wife, Beth. She pitched in 100 percent to make it happen. I used to eat dinner most nights in a corner of the kitchen, at the bar. You know, a raised part of the kitchen counter with a few stools. The TV was usually playing in the background and there were always a few dishes scattered around. If I didn't eat from paper plates it was those pinkish plastic dishes and whatever else was around. When I look back, the place I was eating at looked a lot like the kind of restaurant I wouldn't set foot in if I was starving to death!

"But that all changed with the 'Total Push' idea. From that point on, I had every meal—including breakfast—in the dining room. Up till then it had basically been a place for the kids to do their home-work! I figured my homework—putting on some weight—was more important. Beth did it exactly the way you suggested.''

"How was that?''

"Actually it was a real surprise. I came home from a business trip—I'd flown to Boston—and I was really tired. I had planned to have a cold piece of pizza and maybe a beer and go right to bed. Instead when I walked in the door, she led me to the dining room and I couldn't believe it. No rulers and pencils, no notebooks and cal-culators strewn all over the place. Instead the table was covered with this beautiful white tablecloth. There was a really sensational flower arrangement in the middle and two long ivory-white candles along-side. She even had one of those miniature electric fountains in the center of the floral arrangement. There was music, too—it was a CD of strings playing Strauss waltzes, softly and just in the background.

"The dishes were real china—not expensive but real china. And there were cloth napkins. You know, it's really different from the feel of those paper napkins against your mouth. The food was simple but sensationally good! It was cream of corn soup—one of my favorites. Then we had Lobster Thermidor with plenty of fresh cream and cheese and fried puff potatoes. Everything else was sensational! I must have eaten thousands of calories without even noticing it! What a difference a nice atmosphere makes, Doctor!''

"That's right. You know, when they talk about restaurants, a lot of people say, 'Well, you can't eat the atmosphere!' That's true, but the atmosphere can certainly help you eat! What happened then, Brett?''

"Of course, it wasn't lobster every day. But it was eating in the dining room, instead of that dreary kitchen. I always had flowers on the table, even if it was only a bunch of daisies. I always had music, but easy-listening type music. I even worked out a routine. At break-fast, I usually had something cheerful like songs with a beat. At lunch I went for instrumentals. At suppertime, I really liked the strings, just like the first time.''

"What about eating away from home?''

"If I had to eat with a client, I always steered us to a restaurant with music, plenty of daylight, plants, and good wholesome food. The clients seemed to like it better, too. If I had to eat in the office, I did the same thing—music, flowers, a little tablecloth—everything for the 'total push.' And one more thing. At home, whenever I could, I ate outdoors. We don't have a big backyard but we have a nice terrace. I put out some comfortable tables and chairs and a big umbrella over the table and when the weather is good, I try to eat there at least twice a day. It's amazing what fresh air can do for your appetite!''

"You're right! How did the 'total push' idea work for you?''

Brett tugged at his belt. "I let this belt out two notches in the past couple of months. And I'm up to 122 pounds. That's the most I've weighed in a long time! And most important of all, now I really look forward to mealtime!''

Jeannie had another kind of problem. She had come up against a brick wall and didn't know what to do next. She was tall, dark haired, and attractive and looked much younger than her 34 years. Let her tell about it:

"You know, Doctor, I'm a systems analyst with an industrial consulting company and I have to make a lot of presentations to clients. I don't know how they feel about it, but being so much underweight really was draining away all my self-confidence. It was really important for me to gain weight, and I tried hard to eat and do all the things I should be doing but I kept coming up against one big obstacle.''

"What was that?''

She hesitated a moment and then went on. "I don't know if I should tell you. Maybe you'll laugh when you hear it.''

"Don't worry about that. This is all serious business.''

"Okay. I decided to apply the same techniques of systems analysis that I used every day in my work to my underweight problem. Believe me, it wasn't easy. I made all the lists and did all the charts and I just couldn't put my finger on what was holding me back. Until one day I stumbled on the explanation.

"I had made a list of everything I had eaten for the past month—with the caloric values and amounts of each item."

"But wasn't that a monumental task?"

"It sure was! But I was getting desperate. I knew how dangerous it was to be underweight and yet in spite of everything I was doing, I wasn't gaining as much as I should have been. Well, what I found out was really amazing. It must have been going on all my life and I just wasn't aware of it!

"I was suffering from acute 'BB,' 'LB,' and 'SB.' As a matter of fact, I was on the brink of total 'FB'!"

"Can you be a little more exact?"

Jeannie laughed. "Sure. You know, in the systems business, it's all computers and abbreviations. What I found was that I suffered from acute 'Breakfast Boredom,' 'Lunch Boredom,' and 'Supper Boredom' and I was well on my way to total and absolute 'Food Boredom.' I was eating the same thing over and over and over again. It had gotten to the point that I could sit down to a meal blindfolded and tell you exactly what was on my fork before I bit into it! I was beginning to feel like the famous Cheeseburger Phantom!"

"The *Cheeseburger* Phantom?"

"That's right. That was the man who ate lunch every day for 19 years in the same hamburger place in Los Angeles. He had a cheese-burger, an order of French fries, and a strawberry milk shake every single day, 7 days a week at exactly 12:15 P.M. for 19 years! I never saw a picture of him but I bet he was underweight, too!"

Jeannie took a chart out of her very roomy purse. "Look. Here's my breakfast: 1 bowl of cereal with 1 sliced banana, ¼ cup milk, and 2 teaspoons of sugar. 1 slice of white toast with orange marmalade. One cup of coffee with 2 tablespoons of cream and 1 teaspoon of sugar. I ate that breakfast—with only minor variations—79 percent of the time!"

She rustled around in her purse and took out another chart. "Here's my lunch. In my specialty we would call this a 'Modal' lunch—that means the kind of lunch I ate more often than any other kind: 2 slices of whole wheat bread, 2 slices of luncheon meat, 2 tablespoons of mayonnaise, 1 leaf of lettuce, 1 small bag of potato chips, 8 ounces of a soft drink, 1 small piece of chocolate cake. Can you believe it? I ate this lunch, only varying the kind of luncheon meat, 71.5 percent of the time. By the way, 71.5 percent of the time means that I actually ate it 5 days out of every week. But weekends weren't much better.''

''What do you mean?''

''Well, weekends I usually just sent out for a pizza—62 percent of the time. And sometimes I defrosted a frozen dinner—20.3 percent of the time.''

She blushed slightly. ''I'm sorry to have everything so methodical but that's what helped me find the problem. Now to the solution. What I did was make a list of every possible food that I might like. I didn't leave anything out. That is, I included things like raw fish—in the form of sushi, of course—and snails and tofu, that soybean cake. Then I listed them in order of calories and picked the top 100 food items that had the most calories. Then I distributed them throughout the week so I had to try at least one new food every day. I know that's a lot more trouble than most people would want to go through but I have all the programs working on my computer at the office already. It's easy for me!''

''How did it work out?''

Jeannie smiled from ear to ear. ''Would you believe 9 pounds in two months? And that was without really pushing too hard. I discovered so many great things to eat that I never even imagined existed!''

''For example?''

''Well, Doctor, first of all, let me start by saying that I'm sure not everyone shares my taste. What I love, someone else may hate—and vice versa. But I'd sure recommend that each and every one of your patients try as many new foods as they possibly can. It's an adventure, it's exciting, and it puts on the pounds!''

She took a deep breath and continued. ''First I tried different meats—things that I had never even tasted. I ate goose—it was wonderful and really fattening. Then I tried foie gras—you know, goose liver pâté. The imported version is expensive but the kind that's made here is reasonable and very very caloric. I'd had plenty of lamb chops but I'd never eaten mutton. I tried that and I liked it. It's a different taste. I even tried goat meat because I saw it on the menu a lot when I was in Mexico.''

Jeannie shrugged her shoulders. ''It was all right but I wouldn't fight anyone to eat it again. But it served its purpose. By the time I was two days into this program, I had whipped 'FB' forever. I couldn't wait for my next meal! I looked forward to the surprise and excitement of trying something that I had never eaten before. Instead of a chore, eating was really fun—for the first time in my life.

''I also discovered something amazing. There are so many different foods and dishes that people eat all around us every day that we don't even know about—or are too snobbish to even try. For example, I had fried 'platanos.' Those are the big green bananas—although they aren't really bananas—that you see in the Latin markets. When you slice them and fry them up, they get so delicious—and so fattening— that you can't believe it! I also tried Halvah from the Middle Eastern markets. Not the kind that comes in cans but the homemade types. Wow! That's basically sesame paste with sugar and it tastes great and it really puts the pounds on. And then I tried something I'd always wanted to try—grits. You may not believe it, but I love grits. I eat them for breakfast just like they do in the South. And they pack calories, believe me, especially if you make them the way I like them.''

''How's that?''

''The real old-fashioned way! I'm sure you know what grits are, Doctor. It's dried corn that's ground fine with the bran and the germ taken out. You cook them in water like rice. Then when they get cold you pack them in a square shallow pan and cut them in thick slices. Then you fry the slices in bacon fat and when they're piping hot and aromatic, you serve them covered in hot sugar syrup. Yummy!''

Jeannie's idea was brilliant—and very useful to all of us who want to gain weight. While we may not share her exact tastes, her concept serves two important needs. First, it makes eating interesting and exciting all over again. We can anticipate mealtime again with all the new tastes and textures and discoveries. Second, it gives us the chance to eat more. New foods bring new appetites—and new calories.

Of course we don't have to eat the grits that Jeannie loves so much—or the goat meat that she didn't particularly care for. But if we can make eating exciting and adventurous, we will have made great strides forward. This is the way to start. Take the time—on a day when you're not rushed—to check the items in a large super-market that you may not have noticed before. If anything seems new or unusual to you, ask about it and see what the employees can tell you. Then give it a try. But don't stop there. Ask your friends to suggest unusual foods they may have liked. And by all means, check the local ethnic markets. Ask about the unusual items you may see displayed in the Latin and Chinese and Thai and Vietnamese and Middle Eastern markets—and all the other new and exotic places that have opened up recently. You will be educated, surprised, and delighted, I'm sure. And best of all, you'll gain weight in the process.

To make things easier, here's a list of things that you just might want to begin with:

Middle Eastern: baklava, hummus, halvah, kibbe, bulghur
Chinese: Everything you don't already know. Be brave! Be adventurous!
Japanese: Try the lesser known—and far more exciting—forms of sushi. Go beyond maki and California roll to yet uncharted waters. (Ask about the sushi that is aphrodisiac.) Try the delicious Japanese dumplings known as "gyoza"—and anything else that you come across.
Indian: Try everything! You'll find a lot of calories hidden there.

Latin: I can't even begin to make a list. Just ask any of
the cheerful employees—or customers—to make
suggestions. You'll be amazed at how enthusiastic
they will become—especially if you take food seriously.

These are only places to begin. Use your imagination and ingenuity and you'll be amazed and delighted how much more interesting and enjoyable eating will become.

There's something else that can help us, too. We need to become
"calorie misers." Real-life misers are obsessed with money. They
don't think about very much else and they know the price of everything. These are the folks that count their change down to the last
penny, who know their bank balance to the second decimal point, and
who never spend a nickel if they don't have to. If that's the way they
like to be, we shouldn't criticize them. As a matter of fact, we can
learn from them. Not how to hoard money, but how to hoard *calories.*

Look at it this way. We make as much money as we can, but we
have to spend money to live. If we miss a chance to pick up $20 or
$50 extra, it means that we lose money. Our bank balance gets thinner.

We have to absorb calories to live. And we have to use up
calories to live—remember those 1.5 calories a minute that are being
drained away no matter what we are doing. In real life you can cut
your expenses and save more money. But in a practical sense, you
can't cut down on your physical activity to build up your weight. (If
you try it, you will only make even bigger problems for yourself.)
But what you can do, easily and effectively, is become a "calorie
miser." Don't let one little calorie escape from your grasp. Take
every tiny calorie seriously. Chris learned that early in the game.

"At first I thought it was a joke, Doctor. You know, go chasing
after every little calorie. I mean, what difference can 3 or 4 calories
make in my life? And then I found out."

"What do you mean?"

"I just got out my pencil and paper and did some figuring. I'm a copilot for a major airline and I have a lot of time on layovers to do things like this. I also have a big interest in gaining weight. The airline I work for doesn't impose weight requirements on its pilots and copilots—they have enough problems worrying about the weight of the stewardesses. But I know that if I put on some weight and have a better personal appearance, my chances of moving ahead will be a lot better. You know, we have a lot of contact with the public and that's where appearance counts. Especially if I ever want to move up into management.

"So I did the numbers. Wow! What a surprise! The first calculation was the obvious one. If I can save 3 calories, that's what I lose every 2 minutes of my life—minimum, even if I'm sleeping. But I can lose twice that if I even start to be active. So an extra soda cracker—even one of those little squares—adds at least 12 calories. That's almost 10 minutes of calorie burn-off that I'm replacing. If I can eat an extra cookie—say, a ginger snap—in the course of the day, that's another 25 calories or 20 minutes of burn-off that I'm putting back."

Chris paused a moment. "And then I got to thinking about fat people. Don't they count every calorie? I watch the passengers sometimes—especially the ladies who are overweight. They say things like, 'Oh don't touch that! Two of those have 50 calories!' If they're smart enough to pass 50 calories by, I should be smart enough to grab it and make it part of my program!

"Every time I see a stray calorie go by, I grab it! I munch those nuts we give away to passengers while I'm in the cockpit. I always have some candy or a snack in my pocket. The console of my car sometimes looks like a convenience market with potato chips and tortilla chips and assorted nuts and raisins. I feel that if I'm doing something that allows me to chew and I'm not chewing, then I'm letting myself down."

"How has it worked, Chris?"

"Better than I ever expected. I started off weighing 134 pounds—I'm exactly 6 feet tall."

"That gives you a BMI of about 18½."

"That's right. Now, just by chasing calories—a 'calorie miser,' as you put it—I'm up to 140 pounds in only two months. And remember I have the tremendous disadvantage of eating one day in New York, the next day in Hong Kong, and the third day in Calcutta. If you think that's easy!"

"I'm sure it's not. Tell me more about Calorie Chasing."

"As I mentioned, I have plenty of free time. So I go through all the food lists looking for ways to steal a few extra calories. For example, what you said about cooking pasta 10 minutes instead of 20 minutes to save 25 percent of the calories made an impression on me. I checked through my lists and discovered that red salmon has 18 percent more calories than pink salmon—for exactly the same-size can! I also discovered that there can be an 8 percent difference between different brands of American cheese. The cheese can look alike, it can taste alike, it can seem almost identical, but if you read labels carefully, you get the 8 percent bonus free! Or sometimes the brand with more calories costs less!

"It's the same thing with canned peas. One brand can have 33 percent more calories than another brand—and you'll never know unless you read the label. If you eat the lower-calorie kind, you get just as full, but you won't put on as much weight. The difference is a little less in frozen peas—25 percent less calories with some brands. But 25 percent is nothing to sneeze at. That means for every 4 pounds of weight you can expect with one brand you'll put on 5 pounds with the other—eating exactly the same amount of peas!"

Chris patted his stomach. "It's a little extra work to check up on those calories, but it pays off!"

He's right. It's not hard to snag an extra 900 calories during the course of a week. That will put on an extra ¼ pound a week, or a pound a month—with no extra work and no extra eating. It's the easiest job anyone ever had.

Speaking of easy jobs, here's another way to add pounds without having to eat one mouthful more. Human beings—and animals— have their own biorhythms. Every function of our bodies operates according to its own private internal clock, which is synchronized with the master clock of our organism. That's what we call the "Diurnal Rhythm," or the daily ebb and flow of hormones, enzymes, blood circulation, and all the rest of the vital functions.

For example, the production of cortisol, one of the most important of the cortisone-like hormones of our bodies, is at its lowest level at about 4:00 A.M. That's when we are most sluggish and apathetic. But by the time 9:00 A.M. rolls around, we have plenty of cortisol and we are raring to go. (Well, some of us are, anyhow.) The important point for those of us who want to gain weight is that our body metabolism drops to its lowest during the hours of sleep—say from 11:00 P.M. to about 5:00 A.M. That means we can gain extra weight—from the same number of calories—if we eat something just before going to bed. The midnight snack—or the ten-o'clock snack—has always been the bane of folks who want to lose weight. But for us, it can be a wonderful benefit. You don't have to eat much but be sure to eat something every night before you go to bed. If you have trouble sleeping with a full stomach, just have a couple of crackers with butter and jam or a few cookies. If it doesn't bother you to eat seriously at bedtime, try a piece of cake with ice cream or some cheesecake or a ham sandwich. But no matter what, do your best never to go to bed hungry. A nice high-calorie snack at bedtime is worth its weight in gold the next day. Try it and I'm sure you'll be delighted with the results.

## Chapter Fourteen

# Pure Weight-Gain Pleasure: Exciting Menus and Tantalizing Tidbits

**N**ow it's time for some exciting menus and luscious recipes, enhanced to give us more calories and more flavor at the same time. You'll find the menus easy to put together. Most of them are made up of items you'll find at the local supermarket. (We've added a very few that are a little offbeat just to make life more interesting.)

One of the big questions that keeps coming up on a weight-gain program is "What should I eat?" I know how it is. Sometimes nothing seems to appeal to us. We fall into a kind of gastronomic never-never land, and we tend to take the easy way out. That means a couple of bites of cold pizza that has been sitting on the refrigerator shelf since Saturday night and a swig of soda pop that has gone slightly flat. That's an excellent way to *lose* weight. But to gain weight we need to always have food on our mind. Let's lend a helping hand by listing some sample menus.

You can start off by eating a meal just the way it is presented. After that you can mix and match to your heart's content. You can take the main dish from one meal and switch it with the main dish in another meal. You can do the same thing with the beverages, vegetables, and desserts. If you have, say, 20 meals with an average of 5 dishes in each meal, you will have more possible combinations than the roulette table at Monte Carlo.

Let's start off with some sample breakfasts. These are "idea" breakfasts, of course. If you can't eat everything in each example, eat as much of each item as you can. And if you want second helpings, of course don't hesitate to ask for them. But based on what you know by now, you should be able to construct excellent enhanced breakfasts that will give you a big advantage in your weight-gaining program. Let's start off with some breakfast ideas.

Strawberries and cream
Fried eggs with pork sausages
Raisin toast
Currant jelly
Croissants
Coffee with cream and sugar

Stewed prunes and figs
Pecan pancakes with hot maple syrup
Fresh peach jam
Hot buttermilk biscuits
Coffee with cream and sugar

Applesauce with raisins and walnuts
Fried eggs with fried grits
Bacon
Orange waffles with honey
Coffee with cream and sugar

Peaches and cream
Ham omelet
Rye pancakes★
Cream biscuits★
Fresh plum jam
Coffee with cream and sugar

Stewed mixed dried fruit (peaches, apricots, and pears)
Fried apple rings
Sweet potato waffles with syrup
Broiled ham

* Dishes marked with ★ have recipes in this chapter.

Crackling bread★
Coffee with cream and sugar

Sliced bananas in cream
Grape Nuts cereal
Cheese omelet
Canadian bacon
Doughnuts
Coffee with cream and sugar

That's the basic concept for breakfast. You can mix and match, add anything you want, and introduce endless variations. But the basic principle is to use delicious, high-calorie foods to get your day off to a good start. The key point is to get ahead of that relentless 1.5-calories-a-minute calorie burn-off that constantly works against you.

Now let's see some sample lunch menus. We'll start off with lunches you can make and eat at home—then we'll go on to the eating out and "take-it-with-you" lunch menus.

Avocado cocktail salad★
Fried chicken with cream gravy★
Hash brown potatoes
Buttered peas
Pineapple cream pudding
Coffee milk shake

Cream of mushroom soup
Baked eggs and Canadian bacon on toasted English muffins
    with Hollandaise sauce
Melted cheese sandwiches
Rum custard
Chocolate milk shake

Split pea soup
Barbecued spareribs
Eggplant parmigiana

Creamed celery
Prune pie
Soda pop

French eggs on rice★
Avocado, grapefruit, and cheese surprise salad★
Baked potato with sour cream
French-fried cauliflower
Chocolate peppermint cake
Strawberry milk shake

That's the general idea for lunches at home where you can take the time and effort to pack the maximum amount of calories into each forkful. If you take your lunch to work, you can still enjoy delectable meals and plenty of calories. But there is one thing to keep in mind if you bring your lunch from home. Some take-it-with-you lunches have to be refrigerated or at least kept in a small cooler box. Dishes that contain perishable meats or fish, eggs, or mayonnaise need to be kept cool. If they stay at room temperature for a few hours, they can develop dangerous concentrations of bacteria, and we want to avoid anything like that. These lunch menus are wonderfully tasty meals, but they must be kept cool until the time they are eaten.

To get us off to a good start, here are some excellent high-calorie combinations:

Liver sausage sandwiches with butter and pistachio nuts
Creamy potato salad (in plastic container)
Cole slaw (in plastic container)
Cheese sticks
Fruit cake
Chocolate milk shake from supermarket dairy case (in
    Thermos bottle)

For all the following sandwich spreads, simply combine all the ingredients in a food processor or blend and mix thoroughly.

Special cream cheese peanut butter sandwich spread (½ cup peanut butter, ½ cup mayonnaise, 3 tablespoons pickle or pickle relish)

Cabbage salad with mayonnaise (in plastic container) Remember that raw cabbage helps to slow thyroid activity.

Potato chips

Dried dates

Chocolate-covered graham crackers

Vanilla milk shake from supermarket dairy case (in Thermos bottle)

Special cream cheese nut sandwich spread (¼ cream cheese, ¼ cup mayonnaise, ¼ cup ground walnuts, pecans, cashews, or pistachios, ¼ cup ground raisins)

Shoestring potatoes

Dried prunes

Fried pork rinds

Brownies

Malted milk from supermarket dairy case (in Thermos bottle)

Special ham and relish sandwich spread (2 slices supermarket boiled ham, ½ cup mayonnaise, ¼ cup pickle relish)

Macaroni salad

Onion-flavored rings (snack food)

Dried apricots

Lemon pie (from supermarket—one piece, individually wrapped)

Fruit punch

Special blue cheese and nut sandwich spread (½ cup blue cheese, ½ cup Monterey Jack or other white

cheese, ¼ cup mayonnaise, 1 teaspoon Worcester-
    shire, ¼ cup chopped walnuts or pecans)
Tuna salad with mayonnaise
Tortilla chips
Mixed dried fruits
Canned fudge pudding
Soda pop

The nice thing about sandwiches is that we can load them up
with high-calorie spreads to our heart's content. If we want more
calories, all we have to do is make the spread a little thicker or add
more fat-containing ingredients to the recipe. Here are some excellent sandwich main ingredients, and I'm sure by now you can think
of many more yourself.

Bacon, lettuce, and tomato with mayonnaise
Crabmeat with melted cheese on thickly buttered toast
Sliced cheese and bacon
Chopped hard-boiled eggs and ham
Chopped liver and bacon with added butter★
Blue cheese, cheddar cheese, and bacon
Canned salmon with sour cream
Cheddar cheese, onions, ketchup, cream★
Cheddar cheese, ham, mayonnaise, cream, and spices★
Cream cheese, mayonnaise, and nuts
Cream cheese, mayonnaise, Russian dressing, peanut
    butter★
Cream cheese, butter, and spices★
Chicken salad surprise with capers and celery★
Liver sausage with mayonnaise and spices★
Peanut butter, mayonnaise, and banana, or Raisins or
    Prunes★
Mashed baked beans, mayonnaise, and spices★

Of course, you can use any of the standard ingredients for sandwiches including luncheon meats, roast beef, roast pork, chicken,
turkey, and anything else that you particularly like. But be sure to

add liberal amounts of mayonnaise or butter or margarine to get in as many calories as possible.

These are only a few examples—you will surely be able to think of many more yourself. By the way, you'll notice that mayonnaise figures prominently in many of the recipes, along with peanut butter and butter. That's because it packs so many calories into such a small space. For example, one single tablespoon of mayonnaise or peanut butter or butter can give us about 100 calories. And speaking of butter, if you prefer you can substitute polyunsaturated margarine or oil for butter anywhere in any recipe.

For those of us who have to eat lunch at a restaurant there are some exciting possibilities. Let's analyze that situation for a moment. Restaurant menus don't happen by accident. They are carefully designed by professionals to encourage the customers to order as much as possible and to consume as much as possible. That translates into the biggest possible ''ticket,'' as the customer's bill is known in the trade. The most profitable restaurants are usually the ones which give a lot of food at a relatively reasonable price and encourage massive consumption.* One of their secrets of success is to combine fat with saltiness and sweetness. Why? Well, a reasonable—although not excessive—fat content in dishes provides the quality everyone loves: a pleasant ''mouth-feel.''

The way ice cream is designed is a good example. Ice cream with a generous fat content feels smooth and rich—it has a good ''mouth-feel.'' That's what customers are willing to pay for. Good ice cream is also sweet—but not cloyingly so. It satisfies you without choking you. And although we don't usually think about it consciously, quality ice cream is also fairly salty. That saltiness accentuates the sweet flavor at the same time it tames it and brings it under control.

If we keep those three qualities in mind, the success of the most popular types of mass-market restaurants begins to make sense. Mexican food, for example, provides the perfect combination of those ideal qualities. It has generous amounts of fat—both in the ingredi-

* The ultrafashionable places that give you a tiny portion of food in the middle of a large plate are the exception. Underweight folks *never* go there.

ents and by virtue of the fact that many of the dishes are fried in oil. Mexican dishes also have substantial amounts of salt, which encourages us to eat more to dilute the salt as we are working our way through the meal. A little-known ingredient in commercial Mexican food is sugar—or at least sweetener.* A dash of sugar (or perhaps more than a dash) perks up the taste buds and encourages us to eat more. Incidentally most commercial sausages, including hot dogs, contain a generous dose of sugar.

That's all good news for those of us who want to gain weight. Mexican food is loaded with calories and in a way that makes it fun to eat and makes each mouthful push us onward to the next mouthful. That's particularly true of hot pepper ingredients so prominent in Mexican cooking. Take a bland dish like refried beans. Basically that consists of boiled beans, mashed and fried with added fat and relatively mild spices. But add hot peppers or hot "salsa" (the Spanish word for sauce) to the beans, and everything changes. Suddenly we get into an interesting cycle.

The hot sauce makes the fried beans taste better, but it's also a little irritating to the lining of our mouth. From a medical point of view, a chemical in the hot peppers called capsicum irritates the free nerve endings in the mucous membrane that lines our mouth. It's similar to what happens when you get alcohol in a cut, although much milder. To reduce the mild irritation from the hot sauce, we eat more of the fried bean puree. But that's too bland, and we add more hot pepper. Then it gets hotter than we like! By the time we have it all adjusted, we have consumed quite a bit of beans cooked with fat. Good news for us!

There's another interesting—and little-known—effect of hot peppers that can work to our benefit. As we can all testify, sometimes eating hot peppers directly or in the form of hot sauce is downright painful. The next and obvious question is, if it is painful, why do people do it? Who wants to eat something that hurts their

---

* More than 1000 years ago sugar was first introduced into daily cuisine by the Chinese, who used it not so much as a sweetener, but as a condiment to heighten the taste of other foods.

mouth every time they eat? Strange as it may seem, the answer is found in the old joke. Remember the man who kept banging his head against the wall? One of his friends stopped by and asked him why he was doing it. With a strange look he explained, "Because it feels so good when I stop!"

Well, in the case of hot peppers, it is much more than a joke. The pain caused by the capsicum acting on the lining of the mouth triggers the secretion of certain exotic substances in the brain known as "endorphins." And endorphins are exactly what they sound like—they are chemical substances produced from inside the body (that's why they're called "endo"). The "orphin" part means that they are natural opiumlike chemicals, similar to morphine. So when you eat hot peppers or hot sauce you fire a burst of natural morphinelike chemicals in your brain. That produces a sensation of well-being and euphoria that no other food can begin to duplicate. It's really a food-induced—and completely legal—high. It also relaxes you and makes it easy to take more time to eat in a leisurely manner. When the feeling wears off—in a few minutes—you are eager to bring it back again. And the easiest—and still legal—way to do it is to eat some more hot peppers. But then you have to eat more food to tone down the effect of the hot peppers—and before you know it, you have eaten twice the calories you started out with.

That's why hot sauce and hot peppers can be one of our greatest allies in our effort to gain weight. If we combine them with bland dishes like rice, beans, spaghetti, noodles, and the like, we will end up eating much more than we planned and getting benefits—and feelings—we never even imagined.

But what if you don't like "hot things" on your food? Well, the value of hot peppers (in all their various forms) for gaining weight is so great that it's at least worth a try to get them into our diet. Here's a simple technique that works for almost everyone and gives you the pleasure of the endorphins without the pain.

Get yourself a small bottle of hot pepper sauce—most of them come in those tall, narrow little bottles. Take about half a cup of rice or mashed potatoes or mashed beans and add *one drop* of the hot sauce. Mix it in well and eat the rice or potatoes or beans as you normally would. The next time, add 2 drops—but only 2 drops. As each day goes by gradaully increase the amount of hot sauce you use until you get to a comfortable level. Even a couple of drops will make a difference for you as far as encouraging you to increase your food intake. The idea is not to suffer but to add a bit of zest to your daily diet, increase your consumption of calories, and experience the pleasure of a rush of endorphins. You can also add the hot sauce to soups and stews and anything liquid. Once you begin to enjoy it, you can use it in sauces and many other dishes.

That's why Mexican food is a good choice at lunchtime. Go for the tacos—meat inside rolled-up or folded tortillas. The folded tortillas are usually fried in oil and tacos can be covered with cheese or sour cream—all adding to the caloric benefit. You can also order "chicharrones"—fried pork rinds—which are tasty and loaded with valuable calories. Another good choice is tamales. Contrary to what some people believe, a "hot" tamale rarely exists. (By the way, the singular is "tamal"—"tom-ah." The plural is "tom-ahl-aze.") Tamales are ground corn mixed with meat, vegetables, and spices and then boiled in a wrapper of corn husks or banana leaves. The result is usually quite bland and needs hot peppers to perk it up.

Don't forget about that fabulous dish, guacamole. Basically it is a puree of avocado with spices. But remember that avocado is loaded with calories. A mere half cup of California avocado weighs in at 130 calories. Guacamole goes well inside fried tortillas—tacos—and is even better with just a hint of hot sauce. Remember, the more you eat, the more you gain. Lunch at a Mexican restaurant has most of the ingredients for putting on weight and it's a good choice if you have to eat out at midday.

Italian food is also good—provided you keep some basic principles in mind. If you do it right you can add calories in important amounts while enjoying a first-rate, economical meal. There are just a few key ideas we have to keep in mind.

First of all, we want to add as much olive oil (and/or butter) to the meal as we possibly can. Pick a restaurant that is generous with fats and oils and you will be halfway to your goal. Then be sure to add a certain amount of hot pepper to whatever pasta dishes you choose. Although many people don't realize it, hot pepper is an integral part of the Italian cuisine, and if you ask for it, most good Italian restaurants will rush it to your table. It usually comes in the form of dried flakes that you sprinkle over your spaghetti, macaroni, ziti, or ravioli. Go slowly because the hot pepper flakes are very mild until they absorb some moisture. That brings out their active ingredients, and they start to work for you. So unless you are a veteran user of hot sauce and hot peppers, start off with two or three flakes and proceed step by step. Hot peppers are a wonderful help in gaining weight, but we want to use them prudently and carefully.

Chinese restaurants are also good for lunch provided we take maximum advantage of the benefits they have to offer. The first step is to order as many fried items as possible. Then be sure to include pork dishes on your list instead of chicken. Remember that a 3-ounce serving of chicken averages out to about 115 calories. Three ounces of pork can give you 310 calories. Since it takes the same exertion to chew and swallow the chicken as it does the pork, you get twice the benefit with the same effort. Be sure to use soy sauce liberally since it makes the food that much more appetizing and encourages you to eat more.

At the same time, we shouldn't neglect the hot sauce. Hot peppers are a common ingredient in Chinese food, especially dishes from the province of Szechuan. You'll be surprised and delighted at how much more interesting your favorite Chinese dishes become when you add just a touch of hot pepper flavor to them. But as always, go slow at first. The idea is to bring out the hidden flavors in well-known Chinese recipes—there is no benefit in starting a 4-alarm fire in your tonsils. Once you get used to expanding the flavors of your meals with hot sauce, you may want to slip a little bottle into your pocket or purse so that you have it handy when you eat out.

Oh yes, one final point. What happens if you get a little too much hot sauce and/or hot pepper? How do you put out the fire?

Well, you *don't* throw massive amounts of water in it! Drinking water won't help you that much. There's a more effective solution. Trying sloshing cold milk—or better yet, cream—around your mouth. You can also use ice cream—vanilla is the best. The fat content will neutralize the capsicum in a moment or two, and you won't be any the worse for wear. As a matter of fact, when you get a little too much hot sauce, it triggers an extra spurt of endorphins and you feel an extra "high" a few moments later. That's your compensation.

We can apply the same general principles to any restaurant where we eat regularly. It works the same in Thai, Vietnamese, German, Filipino, and virtually any other restaurant. Just remember to emphasize pork dishes, go for fried foods, add high-fat items whenever possible, and use hot sauce prudently to enhance flavors and stimulate your appetite.

On that subject, there are two more fringe benefits of adding hot sauce to your diet. First, the active ingredients function as an anti-coagulant and give meaningful protection against blood clots. That means, all other things being equal, we should be able to lower our risk of heart attacks and strokes as we increase our intake of hot peppers. A good example is Thailand. That country has one of the highest rates of consumption of hot peppers in the world and one of the lowest incidences of heart attacks and strokes in the world.

The other benefit is in the emotional sphere. Because of its effect in triggering endorphins, if we consume hot peppers over a period of time, we gradually become more optimistic, more active, more energetic, and more self-confident. Apart from all the other benefits, these are just the qualities that encourage us to work harder on our weight-gain program and put on as much weight as we can.

With lunch out of the way, we can go on to some excellent possibilities for dinner menus. Dinner is a key meal since it is the only one we can approach with unlimited time and leisure. The day's work is over, and we can relax from the tensions of the job. Now we can devote ourselves wholeheartedly to one of the most important and enjoyable pastimes in life: eating. Here are some sample choices:

Baked ham with raisin glaze
Broccoli with Hollandaise sauce
French-fried onion rings
Wilted lettuce salad with bacon drippings
Hot Parker House rolls with fresh strawberry jam
Apple brown betty
Fruit punch

Stuffed pork chops
Hash brown potatoes
Buttered noodles
Breaded fried cauliflower (cauliflower polonaise)
Sourdough bread with butter and fresh plum jam
Stuffed dates with nuts*
Milk shake

Cream of mushroom soup
Roast goose with sauerkraut
Hot potato salad
Corn bread with honey
Avocado and grape salad
Rice pudding with chocolate sauce
Malted milk

Chicken loaf
Buttered spinach with egg
Pilaf rice
American fried potatoes
Butterscotch pudding with chocolate-covered graham
    crackers
Date-nut torte
Fruit punch

Baked chicken in cream
Potato dumplings
Buttered lima beans
Lettuce salad with herb mayonnaise

Strawberries with cream
Coffee ice cream
Demitasse coffee

Chicken soup with dumplings
Wiener schnitzel*
Stuffed baked potatoes*
Asparagus with cheese sauce
Apple and raisin salad with curry mayonnaise
Chocolate Bavarian cream*
Bavarian coffee*

You can use these examples to get off to a fast start and later you can expand on them and modify them to suit your tastes. Most of these examples include meat in their menus. There is a good reason for that. Meat is an ''appetite accelerator''—because of its savory qualities it encourages us to eat more. The smell of steaks being barbecued or hamburgers being grilled triggers a whole set of conditioned reflexes in most people. Imagine, for a moment, that you are in a sun-drenched patio on a summer's day with a pair of steaks slowly grilling on a charcoal grill. Think of the tantalizing aroma of the steak and the sizzling of the juices as they fall on the hot coals. Just the thought of it might even make you salivate just a tiny bit. In our war on underweight, we need to use every possible weapon in our arsenal to put on those pounds. Meat is one of those weapons, and it can really help us to gain weight.

However, in all fairness, there are some of us who just don't eat meat. Sometimes it's for ethical reasons and sometimes it's for health reasons, and sometimes it's for personal reasons. But that doesn't matter. We can find a way to gain weight without including meat on the diet. The basic principle is to substitute ''calorie carriers'' for meat. For example, pasta of all sorts—noodles, spaghetti, macaroni, etc.—can ''carry'' important amounts of olive oil, butter, vegetable oil, and high-calorie sauces in addition to the natural calories of the pasta itself. The same applies to rice dishes, including the famous Middle Eastern pilaf in all its wonderful variations. Potatoes offer another opportunity to reinforce the diet with extra calorie value. And eggs are an excellent stand-in for meat in terms of tastiness and caloric value. Here are some typical examples:

## HIGH-OCTANE VEGETARIAN SPAGHETTI AND EGGS

Prepare ½ pound of spaghetti in the usual way—remembering not to cook it too long. Mix with 2 ounces extra virgin olive oil and ½ teaspoon of oregano. Heat 2 cups canned or bottled Hollandaise sauce in double boiler with ½ cup grated Parmesan cheese until cheese melts. Place hot spaghetti on serving plate and garnish with 4 hard-boiled eggs cut into quarters. Pour hot sauce over all. You can sprinkle dried hot peppers prudently over the dish, if you wish.

## QUICK WEIGHT-GAIN CHINESE NOODLE SALAD

Cook 1 pound of egg noodles for about 4 minutes. Rinse under running water and shake dry in colander. Add 4 tablespoons of Chinese sesame oil and 2 tablespoons of first-quality Chinese soy sauce. Refrigerate until well chilled but not stiff.

Serve with the following sauce:

## CHINESE SWEET-SOUR NOODLE SAUCE

6 tablespoons peanut butter

5 tablespoons water

2 tablespoons first-quality Chinese soy sauce

2 tablespoons first-quality Chinese vinegar

8 tablespoons Chinese sesame oil

Hot pepper sauce to your taste

5 tablespoons sugar

½ teaspoon powdered garlic

½ teaspoon powdered onion

Combine all the ingredients in a food processor or blender. Serve the sauce cold on cold noodles or hot on hot noodles.

## QUICK AND EASY EGG-CHEDDAR-RICE BAKE

6 eggs

2 cups cooked rice

3 cups cheddar cheese, grated
2 cups heavy cream
Salt and pepper to taste
Hot sauce to taste—but at least put in a tiny drop or two
¾ cup whole wheat bread crumbs
¼ pound stick of butter

Beat eggs thoroughly and mix with all ingredients except bread crumbs and butter.

Pour into greased baking pan and cover uniformly with bread crumbs. Cut butter into 8 pieces and distribute over top of bread crumbs. Bake for about 35 minutes at 325 degrees or until done.

That's just the beginning. You'll find it easy to enhance your favorite vegetarian dishes simply by increasing the amount of fat in the form of oil, butter, and other shortening. You'll also add calories when you add extra eggs to every recipe that calls for them.

The first thing we need to think about every morning is what we are going to eat that day to put on the weight we need so badly. And the final thing we need to think about every night is what little extra portion of calories we can slip in before our eating day ends. It's so important to keep in mind that 1 calorie at bedtime is worth at least 2 calories the next morning. So it's worthwhile to make a special effort to eat whatever we can before we retire for the night.

The simplest way to slip in a few hundred calories at bedtime is the way kids do all over the country. Have a nice glass of milk and a big piece of cake or pie at bedtime. We can improve on that a bit by opting for a milk shake or a malted milk and choosing a particularly caloric type of cake or pie. Here are some examples that will do the trick:

## BEVERAGES

Hot chocolate (made with milk and cream)*
Enhanced milk shake (various flavors)*
Chocolate-coffee Special*
Almond Secret*

## SNACKS

Chocolate cake with vanilla ice cream
Raisin pie a la mode
Gingerbread with butter cream frosting*
Date-nut torte*
Ice cream roll
Ice cream sundaes—all flavors with nuts and toppings
Peanut butter cupcakes*
Prune cake with whipped cream*

That's only a beginning. Each of us can add dozens of favorite beverages and dishes to this list. The important thing is to "think calories" at bedtime—the time when those calories will do us the most good!

Some of us prefer bedtime snacks that have a stronger flavor, especially on those cool winter evenings. Here's a list of possibilities that will help us to close our day with a few hundred more very useful calories:

Croque-monsieur (French melted cheese sandwiches . . .
    but with a difference)*
High-octane nut and cheese sandwiches*
Cheese-bacon feast*
Sizzling ham sandwiches

For real sandwich fans, there's nothing like a do-it-yourself "torpedo," "grinder," or "submarine" sandwich. Whatever name it goes by, it adds zest to your life and calories to your weight-gain program. The exact recipe is up to you, but a basic list of ingredients—which you can expand endlessly—follows:

Loaf of long crispy Italian or French bread
Extra-virgin olive oil
Italian dressing
Mayonnaise
Ketchup

Mustard
Ham
Bologna
Mortadella
Corn beef
Pastrami
Roast beef (sliced)
Roast pork (sliced)
Roast chicken (sliced)
Roast turkey (sliced)
Assorted cheeses (Asiago, cheddar, provolone, Jack,
    etc.)
Lettuce
Tomato
Onion
Hard-boiled eggs
. . . and whatever else you may think of along the way.

Slice the bread the long way. Line the lower half with lettuce, which keeps the sauces from soaking through to the bread. Then pile on your choice of meats, cheeses, eggs, tomatoes, onions, and sauces and dressings until you get the combination that pleases you. If you can think of anything else that's not on the list, go ahead and pile it on. Then put the top half of the loaf in place, cut the loaf vertically into manageable segments, and enjoy every calorie-rich mouthful.

Putting on the pounds that we so urgently need is a challenge—there's no doubt about that. But if we attack it with persistence, dedication, and determination, we will succeed. And as we lengthen our life, improve our health, and increase our energy, we will be well rewarded for our efforts.

## Chapter Fifteen

# More Fun: Easy Hi-Cal Recipes You Can Make in a Jiffy

This is where we have some fun! Now we can put into practice all the concepts of the Quick Weight-Gain Program. The recipes and menu hints are easy, appetizing, and effective. They will put on the pounds day after day after day. There are just a couple of things we need to keep in mind as we go along. First, this is not a "Nutrition" book in the strict sense of the word. Our number-one goal is to save our lives by putting on pounds and thus cut the risk of premature death and serious disease. Our next goal is to look better as we build up our bodies and develop pleasing lines and attractive proportions.

As you read this chapter you'll notice some interesting things. First, in many places we specify "best-quality." That's especially important because we should try to construct a diet of only the highest-quality foods to make what we eat as exciting and as appealing as possible. That's one of the surest ways to guarantee we will eat as much as we possibly can at every opportunity.

Secondly, almost all the recipes are "Quick-'n'-Easy"—you don't have to spend long hours in the kitchen making recipes from scratch. If we have to cook everything to order, it can make our goal harder to reach, for this reason: If we feel like eating but we know it will take half an hour to whip up a high-calorie dish, we are more inclined to grab something from the refrigerator just to fill that empty space in our stomach. But nine chances out of ten, what we grab will only satisfy our *hunger*. Our goal is more than that. We want to use our hunger as a lever to help us gain weight. On the other hand, if we can throw together a nice high-calorie snack or a little meal in a couple of minutes, we will be more likely to eat that and see the results on the scale the next morning. That's why many of these recipes and menu suggestions are taken from the supermarket shelves and even from the fast-food emporiums.

Third, don't waste a second worrying about fat. For the next six months or so, *fat is our friend.** It will save our lives and protect our health. A few months on a moderately fat diet isn't going to do us any harm. However, years of underweight is guaranteed to sicken and kill us long before our time. Our goal is the *most calories in the shortest possible time* for the next 6 months or so—and that means we *must* include fat in our diet. Then when we're at a safe and healthy weight, we can settle down with a program like *The Save-Your-Life Diet,*[1] the *original* high-fiber diet. But for the moment, it's calories by the thousands that take priority.

Now let's get right down to the fun part and start off with a nice little pasta recipe that's just packed with calories. You'll love it and it will put on pounds fast. And best of all, it's easy to make. It's called "Italian-Fried Ravioli." It's really unique—the pasta gets nice and crisp, almost like Chinese egg rolls. You can make the ravioli from scratch if you want to, but a good supermarket freezer-case ravioli—not canned, of course—will do very well. Just make sure all the ingredients are cooked, as they usually are. Here it is:

## ITALIAN-FRIED RAVIOLI

1 dozen ravioli (if frozen, be sure to defrost them first)

Fry in hot oil until crisp, then drain on a paper towel.

You can serve them with this sauce, if you like:

6 ounces extra-virgin olive oil

1 green pepper, sliced finely (remove the seeds)

2 tomatoes, chopped coarsely

* If you prefer, you can substitute oil for butter in many of the recipes; it's a matter of taste more than anything.

> 4 ounces canned black olives, cut in small pieces
> Pecorino or aged Parmesan cheese for grating
> Salt and pepper to taste

Fry all the ingredients except the cheese until tender—about 15 minutes. Pour over the hot fried ravioli and sprinkle with grated pecorino (or *aged* Parmesan) cheese.

---

Pancakes are great—especially if you dot them with lumps of butter and smother them in syrup. But to avoid "pancake boredom," try the exciting hint of rye flavor in these beauties.

## Rye Pancakes

> 1 cup prepared pancake mix
> 4 tablespoons rye flour
> 3 tablespoons heavy cream

Follow the recipe on the box, but add heavy cream* to the pancake mix instead of milk or water. Serve them hot with a big pat of butter on top of each pancake and plenty of honey or syrup. I can almost taste them now!

---

One of the hazards of ordinary eating is "boredom"—in this case "Bread Boredom." The same old bread in the same old way. These delicious cream biscuits solve that problem and add plenty of calories besides.

## Cream Biscuits

Use any standard biscuit recipe, but substitute heavy cream for milk or water in the recipe.

---

Another way to escape from "bread boredom" is to try this exciting crackling bread. It brightens up our eating in a way we never imagined. And it's simplicity itself to make.

---

* In all these recipes, "heavy cream" means whipping cream—not light cream or Half & Half. The heavy cream adds 50 calories per tablespoon.

## CRACKLING BREAD

Use standard corn bread mix recipe, but add a generous handful of crushed pork rinds or crisp bacon to dough before baking.

After all those high-fiber, lo-cal fruits, the avocado is just what we've been looking for—finally a *fruit* that can pack a caloric wallop. Remember one avocado all by itself gives us about 340 calories if it grew up in California—and a mere 260 calories if it's a native of Florida. (That's because they grow different varieties of avocado in each state. If they grew the same variety in both states, they would have the same caloric value, of course.) Here's a nice way to start a meal or just have a snack during the day.

---

## AVOCADO COCKTAIL

I peeled *California* avocado (firm but not hard), cut into cubes.

I cup California special mayonnaise (½ cup mayonnaise, ½ cup heavy cream, 2 tablespoons chopped anchovy filets, mix well)

Line cocktail cups with crispy lettuce leaves, mix avocado and mayonnaise, and pile into cups. Serve ice cold.

---

Fried chicken is great. No, fried chicken is wonderful! But we can make it even better for us if we add some cream gravy. But that creates a problem. What do we do with all that gravy that's left on the plate after we eat the chicken? Ahh, yes. That's what those cream biscuits were invented for—to sop up all that delicious Cream Gravy. Go to it!

## FRIED CHICKEN WITH CREAM GRAVY

Fry chicken the usual way, using your favorite recipe. (You can even use fast-food or take-out fried chicken for this recipe.)

Make a standard white sauce using these proportions:

5 tablespoons butter
1 tablespoon flour
1 cup heavy cream
Salt and white pepper to taste

Or use a good-quality ready-made white sauce and add ½ cup heavy cream per cup of white sauce. Add 1 tablespoon prepared mustard or Worcestershire sauce per cup of white sauce if you like.

Set out the hot chicken and pour the hot white sauce over it just before serving. And don't forget the biscuits!

---

Eggs and rice go together well, but add a typical French touch and suddenly they seem to have been made for each other. Voilà!

### FRENCH EGGS ON RICE

Use your favorite ready-to-cook rice mixture—it can be rice with macaroni, rice with almonds, Oriental rice—whatever you like best. Prepare it according to the instructions on the package, but when it is good and hot and just before serving, add 6 tablespoons butter or olive oil (whichever you prefer). Mix it well and place a hot poached egg on top of each serving.

Now make a sauce for the eggs. Place ¼ cup of butter in a saucepan and heat slowly until it bubbles and just begins to turn dark. Add a dash of white wine and some freshly ground black pepper. Stir well.

Sprinkle a few small capers over each poached egg and pour the hot browned butter over them immediately.

You can mix any excess butter with the hot rice.

---

Here's our friend the avocado again—this time teamed up with blue cheese and hi-cal macadamia nuts. You'll love it!

### AVOCADO GRAPEFRUIT AND CHEESE SURPRISE SALAD

Cut 2 large, peeled California avocados in half—the *long* way. Remove the seed. Lay each half cut side down and slice vertically. You will end up with attractive half-rings of avocado. Arrange them in circles on a large flat dish. Place a segment of pink grapefruit in the center of each avocado circle. Mix two cups creamed cottage cheese with 1 cup of heavy cream. Place in center of dish.

Pour generous amount of blue cheese salad dressing over avocados and cottage cheese. Sprinkle with chopped macadamia nuts.

This salad works for us two ways—it adds calories and fights the thyroid. And besides that it tastes great! What more could we ask?

## ANTI-THYROID CABBAGE SALAD WITH MAYONNAISE

Remember that cabbage—and certain other vegetables such as *broccoli, cauliflower, cabbage, Chinese cabbage, cress, mustard greens, peppergrass, radish, and roquette*—trap iodine and slow down the activity of your thyroid gland. That means your food is metabolized more slowly and you gain weight faster. Try to include one of these vegetables every day in your diet. But always eat them raw—cooking wipes out any beneficial anti-thyroid activity. This tasty salad has two members of the crucifer family, which should help you twice as much.

> I small head cabbage, finely shredded
> I teaspoon celery seed (not celery *salt*)
> I medium-large white radish, finely shredded

Mix salad ingredients well with the following dressing:

> ½ cup mayonnaise
> ½ cup heavy cream
> 2 tablespoons sugar
> ¼ cup chopped walnuts

Most of the time raw vegetables are the mainstay of our overweight friends. When they need something to munch on, they can always turn to a carrot instead of a cookie. But there are some special raw vegetables that can be our friends, too. Here they are:

## VEGETABLES AGAINST UNDERWEIGHT

Here's another helpful way to slow your thyroid while you are putting on pounds. But to work their magic they have to be eaten *raw*—cooking deactivates the anti-thyroid component. And remember the effect isn't permanent—it only works as long as you continue eating significant amounts of these special vegetables so you don't have to worry about overdoing it. Try this: Have a nice dish of these assorted vegetables handy in the refrigerator to munch on anytime. Include these for sure:

*Broccoli*
*Cauliflower*
*Chinese Cabbage*
*Radish*

Since they don't have much in the way of calories themselves, always cover them with generous amounts of a caloric salad dressing like this one:

## CREAM DRESSING FOR ANTI-THYROID VEGGIES

½ cup heavy cream
4 tablespoons white wine vinegar
1–2 tablespoons horseradish (whole chunk or prepared from a bottle)
Salt and pepper to taste

Put all the ingredients in blender or food processor but do not *overblend* or the cream will turn to butter! Then chill well and keep in refrigerator next to anti-thyroid vegetables.

Now let's turn to one of our biggest allies in the fight against underweight—the mighty sandwich! We all know the story of the famous Earl of Sandwich who didn't want to be disturbed during a card game and so "invented" the sandwich. That must have been interesting news to the Chinese, the folks in the Middle East, and the people of the Caribbean, who had been eating various kinds of sandwiches for at least 10 centuries before the good earl decided not to interrupt his card game. Anyhow, whatsoever name you put on it, the sandwich is an excellent "Calorie Carrier," and here are some fillings that provide the calories. You can make them up beforehand and keep them refrigerated. Then just spread on a slice of bread, slap another slice on top, and you have a plateful of potential pounds ready to be eaten.

Here are a few helpful hints. Your very best bet calorically is presliced white bread because it won't fill you with fiber before the sandwich filling fills you with calories. But you don't have to use it *all* the time. You can use Middle Eastern *pita* bread, south-of-the-border tortillas, Indian *chapatis,* or any other type of bread that strikes your fancy. It's a good idea to try all the different types—we want to avoid menu monotony at all cost.

Sandwiches have another advantage—they are eminently portable. Don't be afraid to pack them up and take them with you. A little insulated bag like they use for baby nursing bottles will keep them cool until you're ready to eat them. And there are some sandwiches—like the famous peanut butter and jelly or peanut butter and pickle relish and similar variations—that don't even need refrigeration or cooling. One little tip. If your sandwiches are going to travel with you, line the bread with a carefully dried leaf of lettuce before you spread on the filling. That will help ''waterproof'' the bread.

One other point. All these sandwich fillings are blended or processed to thoroughly mix the ingredients. But you can decide how much you want them mixed. If you just give them a whirl or two, you'll have a nice chunky spread with the pickles and celery, etc., in recognizable pieces. But let the machine spin for a while and you'll get a smooth, uniform spread with all the flavors thoroughly blended. It's up to you—some days you may feel like eating ''chunky'' and other days you may feel like eating ''smooth.'' It's whatever you feel like—the only thing that matters is getting all those calories down the hatch where they can do their best for you!

Okay, here we go! And be sure to spread these fillings on nice and thick!

## Chopped Hard-Boiled Eggs and Ham

> 4 hard-boiled eggs
> I cup mayonnaise
> 4 slices boiled ham (vacuum packed, from meat case)
> Salt and pepper to taste

Blend or process thoroughly in a blender or food processor, then chill well and keep in refrigerator until ready to spread on bread.

Liver and bacon is another one of those perfect combinations. This
one has added eggs to make it a little more interesting. It is packed
with those calories we love so much.

## CHOPPED LIVER AND BACON WITH ADDED BUTTER

        4 hard-boiled eggs
        6 chicken livers previously fried in a generous amount of
        olive oil
        2 cups mayonnaise
        2 tablespoons Worcestershire sauce
        6 tablespoons butter
        ½ cup crisp fried bacon
        Salt and pepper to taste
Blend or process thoroughly in a blender or food processor, then
chill well and keep in refrigerator until ready to spread on buttered
bread.

Onions, cheese, and tomato sauce—on a nice slice of fresh white
bread. That's real eating!

## CHEDDAR CHEESE, ONIONS, KETCHUP, CREAM

        I cup cheddar cheese (cut into small chunks)
        I cup heavy cream
        5 tablespoons Worcestershire sauce
        2 tablespoons ketchup
        ½ small onion (preferably mild—except for onion fanatics)
        Salt and pepper to taste
Blend or process thoroughly in a blender or food processor, then
chill well and keep in refrigerator until ready to spread on bread.

This is another ideal blending of flavors—with barbecue flavor
included in the bargain.

## CHEDDAR CHEESE, HAM, MAYONNAISE, CREAM, AND SPICES

> 1 cup cheddar cheese (cut into small chunks)
> 4 slices boiled ham (vacuum packed, from meat case)
> 2 cups mayonnaise
> 1 cup heavy cream
> Barbecue spice mix from the spice shelf in the supermarket

Blend or process thoroughly in a blender or food processor, then chill well and keep in refrigerator until ready to spread on bread. Simple, elegant, and loaded with calories—that's what we like!

---

Smooth is the word for this combination but the Russian dressing gives it just that little zing that makes you want to ask for seconds.

## CREAM CHEESE, MAYONNAISE, RUSSIAN DRESSING, PEANUT BUTTER

> 1 cup cream cheese
> ¼ cup mayonnaise
> ¼ cup Russian dressing
> 1 cup peanut butter

Blend or process thoroughly in a blender or food processor, then chill well and keep in refrigerator until ready to spread on bread. Excellent on cocktail rye bread or pumpernickel.

---

Here's a filling that's easy, but not too easy, and spicy but not too spicy. You'll enjoy it.

## CREAM CHEESE, BUTTER, AND SPICES

> 1 cup cream cheese
> ¼ cup butter
> 1–2 tablespoons mixed herbs (choose the selection you prefer from the premixed herbs on the spice shelves of your supermarket)
> 1 tablespoon prepared mustard (Dijon, yellow, brown—whatever appeals to you most)

Blend or process thoroughly in a blender or food processor, then chill well and keep in refrigerator until ready to spread on bread.

Now you can try chicken with a hint of the Far East but friendly and familiar—and delicious!

## CHICKEN SALAD SURPRISE WITH CAPERS AND CELERY

¾ pound of chicken breasts, boned
I cup mayonnaise
4 tablespoons capers
I teaspoon celery seed
¾ teaspoon best-quality curry powder
Salt and pepper to taste (be careful! Some curry powder already has plenty of salt!)

Blend or process thoroughly in a blender or food processor, then chill well and keep in refrigerator until ready to spread on bread.

We tend to take liver sausage for granted—something that goes in our lunch box. But in France it has another name: pâté de foie. If you think about it, it's really an elegant combination of liver combined with delicate spices. Try this version of pâté de foie.

## LIVER SAUSAGE WITH MAYONNAISE AND SPICES

I cup liver sausage
½ cup mayonnaise
¼ teaspoon nutmeg (freshly ground if possible)
Pinch of ground cloves
2 tablespoons butter

Blend or process thoroughly in a blender or food processor, then chill well and keep in refrigerator until ready to spread on bread.

Although the "peanut" is not a nut and "peanut butter" is not butter, it's still a wonderful way to put on pounds while we enjoy what we're eating. This combination brings out the flavor of the banana at the same time that it accentuates that special fresh peanut aroma.

## PEANUT BUTTER, MAYONNAISE, AND BANANA

I cup peanut butter

½ cup mayonnaise

½ cup very ripe banana (the riper the banana, the higher the sugar content, and the better the taste)

2 tablespoons butter

Blend or process thoroughly in a blender or food processor, then chill well and keep in refrigerator until ready to spread on bread.

You can add to this recipe ½ cup of raisins or pitted prunes. It will only make it better—and more caloric.

---

Who ever heard of a baked bean sandwich? Well, we have, and here it is! If you like baked beans, you'll love this combination that you can eat anywhere, anytime. It has all the calories you could wish for!

## MASHED BAKED BEANS, MAYONNAISE, AND SPICES

I can pork and beans (or vegetarian baked beans if you want to avoid the meat)

½ cup mayonnaise

¼ cup chili sauce or seafood cocktail sauce

I teaspoon celery seed

2 sweet pickles

4 tablespoons butter

Blend or process thoroughly, then chill well and keep in refrigerator until ready to spread on bread.

---

Cheese and bacon are always welcome, but with the extra zing of blue cheese, this sandwich could win a prize. You'll really be happy with it.

## BLUE CHEESE, CHEDDAR CHEESE, AND BACON
¾ pound cheddar cheese, sliced
½ pound blue cheese in small chunks
1½ cups mayonnaise
1 cup broken pieces of crisp bacon
4 tablespoons butter

Blend or process thoroughly, then chill well and keep in refrigerator until ready to spread on bread.

---

The salmon is a noble fish and a little bit of sour cream and some capers bring out its special qualities. Try it on rye bread and I think you'll agree it's something special.

## CANNED SALMON WITH SOUR CREAM
1 can red salmon (7¾-ounce size)
1 cup sour cream
½ cup capers
3 tablespoons lemon juice
2 tablespoons butter
3 drops hot sauce (if you feel daring)

Blend or process thoroughly, then chill well and keep in refrigerator until ready to spread on bread.

If you think you picked a winning number in the lottery, you can substitute two cans of *smoked* salmon for the regular salmon. On second thought, considering the price of *smoked* salmon, better wait until you know for sure.

---

Now let's move on from a sandwich to a snack. Here's a nice little hi-cal snack, something that used to be called, in the old days, a "sweetmeat." You can drop a big handful of these into a plastic sandwich bag and slip them into your pocket or purse. They are tasty to munch on, a lot better than candy bars (not to mention cheaper), and they are loaded with calories.

## STUFFED DATES WITH NUTS

Take a dozen big juicy dates and remove the seeds. Select the kind of ready-made cake frosting mix you like the best—chocolate, vanilla, etc. Take a cup of frosting mix and add ½ cup of chopped nuts—walnuts, macadamias, pecans, whatever appeals to you. Mix thoroughly. Make a slit in each date and carefully stuff with the mixture. If you like, you can also add raisins or chopped, crystallized ginger to the frosting mix. Whenever you feel like a snack, pop one of these luscious morsels into your mouth!

---

Every country has its specialty—and even some cities have theirs. Here's the specialty of a very special city—Vienna. It's a veal cutlet made the way they do it in Vienna. That's why it's called "Wiener schnitzel," or a "Vienna cutlet." Our version is a variation that is easier to make and just as easy to eat! The Quick Weight-Gain Program version is called "Kaiserschnitzel"—the "Kaiser's cutlet." That's because it's more elegant, richer, and of course, has more calories. It's quick and easy to make and you'll really enjoy it while it puts on the pounds.

## "KAISERSCHNITZEL"

Have the butcher prepare as many veal cutlets as you want cut about ¾ of an inch thick. Then ask him to pound them until they are nice and thin—about 6 inches by 6 inches in size. At mealtime, dip each cutlet into flour and fry in ¾ cup butter until they are browned well on each side. Then put them in the oven to keep them hot while you are making the sauce.

Don't worry—preparing the sauce is as easy as pie. Just add 1 cup of sour cream that you have kept at room temperature for about an hour to the butter and juices left in the frying pan. Heat it slowly and carefully (so it doesn't curdle) and add a little bit of lemon juice to make it not quite so thick. When it's good and hot, pour it over the veal cutlets and serve right away.

---

Although they have a bad reputation among people who want to lose weight, potatoes aren't really ideal for those of us who want to gain weight. They are full of fiber and fill us up too fast. But potatoes are excellent "Calorie Carriers." If you fry them, they soak up the fat like little starchy sponges. And if you stuff them, they suddenly become very interesting to people like us who want to put on the pounds. You can stuff potatoes with all different kinds of delectable combinations—this recipe is only one possibility, and you can think of many more.

### STUFFED BAKED POTATOES

Bake potatoes until they are completely cooked—½ hour to 1 hour, depending on the size, oven, and moisture content. Then cut them in half, scoop out the inside, and while still hot mash together with ½ cup ready-made white sauce mixed with ½ cup heavy cream and ½ cup melted butter. Add 1 cup shredded cheddar cheese and ½ teaspoon celery seed. (We use celery seed instead of celery sometimes since celery is high in fiber and tends to fill us up too fast. The seeds give the special celery flavor but are not filling.) If you like, you can add ½ cup of peanut butter to the mixture along with or instead of the cheese. You can also add small pieces of chopped Vienna sausages. Put the potato mixture back into the potato skins and return to the oven to heat thoroughly. Serve sprinkled with paprika to give a nice color.

---

Asparagus is a nice vegetable since it has an affinity for cheese—a nice source of calories. Let's whip up a mouthwatering sauce that will help our cause.

### ASPARAGUS WITH CHEESE SAUCE

Take a cup of ready-made white sauce and mix it with 1 cup of heavy cream. Add ½ cup of finely grated Swiss or Gruyère cheese while carefully heating over a low flame (you can use a double boiler if you like). Add 6 tablespoons butter and ½ cup finely chopped canned mushrooms. Pour over hot fresh, canned, or frozen cooked asparagus.

---

Apples don't offer much in the way of calories, but they are delicious and make us want to eat more. That's why they are excellent "Calorie Carriers." In this recipe, they carry nuts and raisins and mayonnaise—all loaded with the calories we love so much!

## APPLE AND RAISIN SALAD WITH WALNUTS AND CURRY MAYONNAISE

Take the cores out of 2 peeled apples. Cut the apples crosswise to get apple rings about ½ inch thick. Arrange them one layer thick on a flat plate. Put a handful of raisins mixed half and half with shelled walnuts on top of each apple ring. Cover the apples and raisins with a generous amount of the following dressing:

I cup mayonnaise

I cup heavy cream

2 tablespoons best-quality curry powder

4 tablespoons sugar

Mix thoroughly in a large bowl.

---

## CHOCOLATE DREAM CREAM CAKE

Here's a nice easy way to add calories and the nice thing is that you can adapt it to almost any kind of cake. We'll use a chocolate cake for this example.

Take a standard 2-layer chocolate cake—it can be made from a mix or bought from a bakery or market. With a spatula carefully lift up the top layer a section at a time and fill with this mixture. Then cover the top and sides with the same mixture.

¾ cup butter

4 cups powdered sugar

8 tablespoons heavy cream

I teaspoon vanilla extract (use *real* vanilla only)

6 tablespoons cocoa powder

Put all ingredients in a food processor and process slowly and carefully until smooth. You can vary the flavor by adding powdered coffee, almond extract instead of vanilla, crushed almonds, or anything else that appeals to you. The basic idea is that most ready-made cakes don't have as many calories in them as we really can use. So if we add an extra layer of frosting and filling, we get the extra flavor—and the extra calories—at the same time.

There is no reason why we can't recruit even our humble cup of coffee to fight on our side in the battle against underweight. Try this version. It's full of good calories and you may even find that it's habit forming!

## Bavarian Coffee

Make a cup of strong coffee—instant is all right but use plenty of coffee powder. Mix with the same amount of Half & Half cream. Add ½ teaspoon vanilla extract (use *real* vanilla only). Serve piping hot, but only fill the cup ¾ of the way. Then cover with a thick layer of very sweet whipped cream (it can be cream from an aerosol can, but make sure it is real cream and not an imitation). Then sprinkle grated chocolate over the top.

If you want an occasional change from coffee, try this chocolate version. It's superb!

## Hot Chocolate

Make hot chocolate in the usual way but use heavy cream instead of milk. Heat carefully and add the cocoa powder according to instructions on the container. Then fill the cup or glass only ¾ of the way. Top with very sweet whipped cream and grated chocolate as in Bavarian coffee.

If there is one food item that seems almost tailor-made for gaining weight, it is the milk shake. Since it is liquid, it goes down fast and easy. It is both sweet and cold—and that makes it even more attractive. Add to that the fact that it comes in dozens of different flavors, which makes it easy for everyone to find just what they want in a cool frosty milk shake. From our special point of view as calorie hunters, the milk shake lets us add plenty of calories without really noticing their most welcome presence.

The milk shake exists in many dozens of countries around the world. Sometimes it appears as a "malted milk" when malted milk powder is added. In Spanish-speaking countries it is called a "batido." If we stretch our imagination a bit we can almost see a distant relative of the milk shake in the Italian "cappuccino" version of espresso coffee.

Here's an old favorite version of the milk shake that will move us that much closer to our weight-gain goals.

## CLASSICAL CHOCOLATE MALTED MILK ("CHOCOLATE MALT")

    ¾ cup ice-cold heavy cream
    ¼ cup ice cold milk
    ¼ cup chocolate syrup (best-quality)
    1–2 tablespoons malted milk powder (use more if you like the "malted" taste, less if you like it less)
    2 big scoops of premium-quality chocolate ice cream (use premium-quality because it has more butterfat and thus more calories)

Put all ingredients in blender and blend until smooth. Serve with a spoon and a straw.

You can increase the taste appeal by varying the flavors of the ingredients and the ice cream you use. Some possibilities are strawberry, chocolate-chip, banana, and the full range of ice cream flavors found at your local ice-cream palace. Just be sure to maintain the proportions of cream to milk so that you get all the calories you deserve.

---

A lot of people in this world like coffee. A lot of people like chocolate. And almost everyone enjoys being present at the happy marriage of coffee and chocolate. If they can add a few hundred extra calories at the same time, so much the better.

Here's a fine recipe:

## CHOCOLATE-COFFEE WEDDING

> I cup strong, hot coffee (espresso might be good here if you really love coffee)
>
> I cup whipped cream (whipped cream in an aerosol can is okay—if it's *real* whipped cream)
>
> 1/8 cup chocolate syrup (best-quality)
>
> 1/4 teaspoon vanilla extract (best-quality)

Dissolve the chocolate syrup in the coffee. Add the vanilla extract. Stir the whipped cream vigorously into the mixture. This is great hot or cold. If you want it cold, add a good slug of crushed ice and serve in a tall glass. It goes well with a couple of cookies on the side.

Almonds have a lot of special qualities, and one of those can help us in our campaign. For centuries almond-based milk drinks were used by Indian tribes in Latin America for medicinal purposes. Almond flavoring seems to settle the stomach and allow us to eat more before we really get full. That's one of the secrets of this delicious drink—the "Almond Secret."

## ALMOND SECRET

> 3 cups heavy cream, ice cold
>
> 1/4 cup milk, ice cold
>
> 1/2 cup crushed ice
>
> 4 tablespoons sugar
>
> I teaspoon almond extract (best-quality)
>
> 2 big scoops vanilla ice cream—premium-quality

Spin all ingredients in a blender until smooth. Serve with crushed, toasted almonds on top.

Ginger is another one of those spices that was used for centuries as a medicine. It can still work its magic as it helps us to eat more without getting full. Gingerbread begs for a nice buttercream frosting, and here's the recipe.

## GINGERBREAD WITH BUTTERCREAM FROSTING

Take a nice ready-made gingerbread cake, or even some ''Ginger-bread Men,'' and cover it (or them) generously with the following frosting. The frosting makes the gingerbread taste better—or, depending on how you look at it, the gingerbread makes the frosting taste better! But any way you look at it, it's plenty more calories!

---

## BUTTERCREAM FROSTING

¾ cup butter

4 cups powdered sugar

8 tablespoons heavy cream

I teaspoon vanilla extract (use *real* vanilla only)

6 tablespoons cocoa powder (optional—for chocolate lovers)

---

''Torte'' means cake, and date-nut torte is a wonderful dish. But if you don't want to bake it from scratch, here's an excellent substitute.

## DATE-NUT TORTE-ROLL

Get a ''date-nut roll''—most supermarkets have them in cans. Cut the roll into disks about 1½ inches thick and cover with a nice thick layer of coconut cream frosting. Here's the recipe:

6 ounces cream cheese

4 cups powdered sugar

1½ teaspoons vanilla extract

I cup ready-made sweetened grated coconut (from the supermarket)

Mix well.

Dates have plenty of calories, nuts have plenty of calories, and coconut has plenty of calories. We really couldn't hope for more!

---

One of our most loyal friends in our weight-gaining program is peanut butter. One tablespoon has about the same calories as a tablespoon of oil or butter. That means that anywhere we can slip in some peanut butter our caloric total takes a great leap forward. Here we can let peanut butter work its magic on cupcakes.

## Peanut Butter Cupcakes

Purchase any kind of cupcakes—frosted or plain. Then refrost them with the following mixture:

> ½ cup peanut butter
> 8 cups powdered sugar
> 8 tablespoons butter
> ¼ teaspoon vanilla extract
> ¾ cup heavy cream

Mix in a food processor until smooth. Add more or less cream to give you the consistency you prefer. Spread lavishly on cupcakes. Place two (or three) whole shelled walnuts on top of each cupcake.

---

As we have seen, any dried fruit is loaded with concentrated calories. Prunes are no exception and we can turbocharge those calories even more if we put our minds to it. Try this one.

## Prune Cake with Whipped Cream

You can use a ready-made prune cake or bake one from a mix. But be sure to cut it into two layers from side-to-side. Spread sweetened whipped cream abundantly between the layers, and then scatter chopped, pitted dates over the whipped cream. Do the same on the top of the cake. The combination of dried prunes, dried dates, and whipped cream makes for plenty of mouthwatering calories that get us ever closer to our goal.

---

There's something about cheese and bacon that goes together perfectly. Maybe it's the texture, maybe it's the smoky flavor of the bacon and the bland flavor of the cheese. But whatever it is, it's a perfect way to add calories and have a nice snack at the same time. Here's a good example:

### CHEESE-BACON FEAST

Butter a nice slice of bread generously. (You can also do this with a big buttery croissant—even more calories!) Cover with 2 slices of your favorite cheese—cheddar is fine here. Then take 4 strips of fried bacon and lay on top of the cheese. Place it all under the broiler until the cheese melts under and around the bacon. Enjoy anytime.

---

There's another type of cheese sandwich that gets its supercharged calories from another source. It's the "High-Octane Nut and Cheese Sandwich." Here's the way to make it:

### HIGH-OCTANE NUT AND CHEESE SANDWICHES

Take a slice of fresh bread and cover it liberally with a layer of butter. Then add two layers of cheddar cheese. Cover the cheese with shelled walnuts or pecans or pieces of macadamia nuts. Top with another slice of buttered bread. Dip the entire sandwich into a well-beaten egg and gently lower it into a fryer (or frying pan) full of hot olive oil or butter. Fry until brown on one side, then turn and brown on the other side. Make sure you cook it long enough to thoroughly melt the cheese. Quick and easy and delicious!

---

No one knows why these delectable sandwich creations are called "Croque-Monsieur"—but it doesn't really matter. What does matter is the taste—and the calories—they bring to us. Here's the basic recipe.

### CROQUE-MONSIEUR

Take a nice slice of fresh bread and cover it liberally with butter—or olive oil. Then spread some tasty mustard on top. It can be French Dijon or brown German or plain old yellow mustard—that's a matter of taste. Then a thick slice (or two thin slices) of best-quality Swiss cheese and finally a slice of smoked or boiled ham and another slice or two of Swiss cheese.

Now we come to a decision. We can put that combination under a broiler and let it heat until the ham is hot and the cheese is melted. That's a great sandwich! Or we can go one step further.

Spread more butter on top of the last layer of cheese, then more mustard on top of that. Then another slice of bread. At this point it's a good idea to hold the sandwich together with a couple of toothpicks for what is about to happen next. (Be sure to take those toothpicks out before you bite into the sandwich. They are "toothpicks," not "gumpicks.")

Gently lower the entire sandwich into a fryer (or frying pan) full of hot olive oil or butter. Fry until brown on one side and then turn over and brown the other side. Make sure you cook it long enough to thoroughly melt the cheese.

A few French pickles—known as "cornichons"—on the side turn this sandwich into a "feastwich." And the calories are there in abundance to help us as well.

These are only a few suggestions to make our campaign to gain weight as successful as possible. If we think calories every minute of the day, we will reach our goal quickly and enjoyably.

Bringing ourselves up to normal weight means a lot more than just improving our appearance. It brings us three important advantages: more energy, better health, and a happier life. Most important of all, it extends our lives so that we have many more years to enjoy what we have accomplished.

Every morning when you wake up, decide to consume as many calories as you possibly can. Plan your menu and eat your meals as if your life depended on it—*because it does*.

Following this chapter you will find a special section, "Basic Principles of Weight Gain." Keep it handy and refer to it at least once a day. You'll find that it will help maintain you right on track with your weight-gain program by constantly keeping the most important concepts at the forefront of your mind.

I wish you the very best success and satisfaction in reaching your goal. Your success is my success and your happiness is my happiness. Remember that I will be happy to hear from you at the following address:

Dr. David Reuben, MD
The Harold Matson Co.
276 Fifth Avenue
New York, N.Y. 10001

# Something to Save: Basic Principles of Weight Gain

**H**ere are 10 Basic Principles of Weight Gain. They summarize some of the most important concepts of this book. Keep them handy so you can refer to them as you put on those pounds. And keep them with you from now on so that you can use them in the future. Good luck!

1. **THERE ARE ONLY 24 HOURS IN A DAY, AND YOUR BODY BURNS UP CALORIES AS EACH MINUTE GOES BY**—even if you don't lift a pencil. If you use as many of those minutes as reasonably possible to absorb calories, you can gain weight. If you waste time on foods that don't give you fair caloric value, you'll have a harder time gaining those pounds.

2. **EACH OF US WAKES UP EVERY MORNING WITH A CERTAIN LIMITED "APPETITE POTENTIAL."** That is, we can only eat so much each day before we get full and can't eat another bite. If we squander our appetite potential on food and drinks that fill us without giving us the calories we need, we may never gain weight—and we can actually lose ounces day by day. So before you eat or drink, ask yourself this: "Is what I am about to consume going to help me reach my goal of putting on pounds?" If not, *don't eat it* but substitute something else that *will* add calories.

3. **DON'T DRINK ANY WATER IF YOU CAN HELP IT**—drink abundant liquid that contains calories instead.

4. **TAKE YOUR EATING SERIOUSLY.** Sit down at mealtime and eat—methodically and systematically. Don't rush but don't eat too slowly. Munch your way from start to finish. For those of us who want to gain weight, eating is always serious business.

5. **USE "WEIGHT-GAIN STRATEGY."** Whenever you are going to eat something, stop a moment to think if there is something else that will give you more calories for the same size, weight, and bulk of food. Avoid foods that have low fat content.

6. **TAKE ADVANTAGE OF THE TECHNIQUE OF "BONUS CALORIES."** It's almost like playing a game where you are always the winner. All you have to do is read every label on everything you buy and look for those extra calories where you least expect them. Do this every day, and you will gradually develop an eagle eye for ''hidden'' calories.

7. **ALWAYS USE "ENHANCED" RECIPES.** Those are recipes that are packed with extra calories that are ''invisible.'' Those are calories that add pounds—but you won't even know they are there. And all these dishes are a pleasure to eat—they are loaded with taste appeal and flavor. The best part is that many of the enhanced recipes take hardly any effort at all. If you work or just don't have the inclination to do a lot of cooking, you can follow the simple instructions and really increase the calories of standard supermarket foods without any inconvenience.

8. **MAKE EVERYTHING THAT YOU EAT PLAY THE ROLE OF "CALORIE-CARRIER."** Add fat and/or sugar to every dish that can absorb it. If you ''piggyback'' calories onto your favorite dishes, you'll find that they take the same effort to eat but the results will be sensational.

9. **ALWAYS CARRY SOMETHING TO EAT WITH YOU TO TAKE ADVANTAGE OF ODD MOMENTS TO ADD A FEW CALORIES**—especially in case you are late, or miss a meal.

10. **NEVER GO TO BED HUNGRY!** Eat at night—every night! When you're asleep, your metabolic rate is slowest. If you eat exactly the same amount at 10 o'clock in the morning and 10 o'clock at night, you will gain more weight from the night feeding!

# Appendix
# Calculating Your Body Mass Index—
# The Easy Way

The Body Mass Index, or "BMI," is a very useful tool for keeping track of our progress. It tells us if we are still underweight or approaching our normal weight. The calculation is simplicity itself but I've made it even easier by doing most of the work ahead of time. This is all you have to do:

1. Go to chart 1, which shows your body weight in pounds and kilos. Select your body weight in kilos and write that number down.
2. Then go to chart 2 and find your height in inches. Look across to the right until you find the Body Surface Area that corresponds to your height. Write that number down.
3. Then divide the bigger number by the smaller number. That number—which should be between 15 and 25—is your Body Mass Index, or BMI.

   The full explanation of the Body Mass Index and its significance are in chapter 1.

# CHART 1
## WEIGHT IN KILOS

| Weight in Pounds | Weight in Kilos | Weight in Pounds | Weight in Kilos |
|---|---|---|---|
| 50 | 22.73 | 80 | 36.36 |
| 51 | 23.18 | 81 | 36.82 |
| 52 | 23.64 | 82 | 37.27 |
| 53 | 24.09 | 83 | 37.73 |
| 54 | 24.55 | 84 | 38.18 |
| 55 | 25.00 | 85 | 38.64 |
| 56 | 25.45 | 86 | 39.09 |
| 57 | 25.91 | 87 | 39.55 |
| 58 | 26.36 | 88 | 40.00 |
| 59 | 26.82 | 89 | 40.45 |
| 60 | 27.27 | 90 | 40.91 |
| 61 | 27.73 | 91 | 41.36 |
| 62 | 28.18 | 92 | 41.82 |
| 63 | 28.64 | 93 | 42.27 |
| 64 | 29.09 | 94 | 42.73 |
| 65 | 29.55 | 95 | 43.18 |
| 66 | 30.00 | 96 | 43.64 |
| 67 | 30.45 | 97 | 44.09 |
| 68 | 30.91 | 98 | 44.55 |
| 69 | 31.36 | 99 | 45.00 |
| 70 | 31.82 | 100 | 45.45 |
| 71 | 32.27 | 101 | 45.91 |
| 72 | 32.73 | 102 | 46.36 |
| 73 | 33.18 | 103 | 46.82 |
| 74 | 33.64 | 104 | 47.27 |
| 75 | 34.09 | 105 | 47.73 |
| 76 | 34.55 | 106 | 48.18 |
| 77 | 35.00 | 107 | 48.64 |
| 78 | 35.45 | 108 | 49.09 |
| 79 | 35.91 | 109 | 49.55 |

| Weight in Pounds | Weight in Kilos | Weight in Pounds | Weight in Kilos |
|---|---|---|---|
| 110 | 50.00 | 143 | 65.00 |
| 111 | 50.45 | 144 | 65.45 |
| 112 | 50.91 | 145 | 65.91 |
| 113 | 51.36 | 146 | 66.36 |
| 114 | 51.82 | 147 | 66.82 |
| 115 | 52.27 | 148 | 67.27 |
| 116 | 52.73 | 149 | 67.73 |
| 117 | 53.18 | 150 | 68.18 |
| 118 | 53.64 | 151 | 68.64 |
| 119 | 54.09 | 152 | 69.09 |
| 120 | 54.55 | 153 | 69.55 |
| 121 | 55.00 | 154 | 70.00 |
| 122 | 55.45 | 155 | 70.45 |
| 123 | 55.91 | 156 | 70.91 |
| 124 | 56.36 | 157 | 71.36 |
| 125 | 56.82 | 158 | 71.82 |
| 126 | 57.27 | 159 | 72.27 |
| 127 | 57.73 | 160 | 72.73 |
| 128 | 58.18 | 161 | 73.18 |
| 129 | 58.64 | 162 | 73.64 |
| 130 | 59.09 | 163 | 74.09 |
| 131 | 59.55 | 164 | 74.55 |
| 132 | 60.00 | 165 | 75.00 |
| 133 | 60.45 | 166 | 75.45 |
| 134 | 60.91 | 167 | 75.91 |
| 135 | 61.36 | 168 | 76.36 |
| 136 | 61.82 | 169 | 76.82 |
| 137 | 62.27 | 170 | 77.27 |
| 138 | 62.73 | 171 | 77.73 |
| 139 | 63.18 | 172 | 78.18 |
| 140 | 63.64 | 173 | 78.64 |
| 141 | 64.09 | 174 | 79.09 |
| 142 | 64.55 | 175 | 79.55 |

| Weight in Pounds | Weight in Kilos | Weight in Pounds | Weight in Kilos |
|---|---|---|---|
| 176 | 80.00 | 209 | 95.00 |
| 177 | 80.45 | 210 | 95.45 |
| 178 | 80.91 | 211 | 95.91 |
| 179 | 81.36 | 212 | 96.36 |
| 180 | 81.82 | 213 | 96.82 |
| 181 | 82.27 | 214 | 97.27 |
| 182 | 82.73 | 215 | 97.73 |
| 183 | 83.18 | 216 | 98.18 |
| 184 | 83.64 | 217 | 98.64 |
| 185 | 84.09 | 218 | 99.09 |
| 186 | 84.55 | 219 | 99.55 |
| 187 | 85.00 | 220 | 100.00 |
| 188 | 85.45 | 221 | 100.45 |
| 189 | 85.91 | 222 | 100.91 |
| 190 | 86.36 | 223 | 101.36 |
| 191 | 86.82 | 224 | 101.82 |
| 192 | 87.27 | 225 | 102.27 |
| 193 | 87.73 | 226 | 102.73 |
| 194 | 88.18 | 227 | 103.18 |
| 195 | 88.64 | 228 | 103.64 |
| 196 | 89.09 | 229 | 104.09 |
| 197 | 89.55 | 230 | 104.55 |
| 198 | 90.00 | 231 | 105.00 |
| 199 | 90.45 | 232 | 105.45 |
| 200 | 90.91 | 233 | 105.91 |
| 201 | 91.36 | 234 | 106.36 |
| 202 | 91.82 | 235 | 106.82 |
| 203 | 92.27 | 236 | 107.27 |
| 204 | 92.73 | 237 | 107.73 |
| 205 | 93.18 | 238 | 108.18 |
| 206 | 93.64 | 239 | 108.64 |
| 207 | 94.09 | 240 | 109.09 |
| 208 | 94.55 | 241 | 109.55 |

| Weight in Pounds | Weight in Kilos | Weight in Pounds | Weight in Kilos |
|---|---|---|---|
| 242 | 110.00 | 247 | 112.27 |
| 243 | 110.45 | 248 | 112.73 |
| 244 | 110.91 | 249 | 113.18 |
| 245 | 111.36 | 250 | 113.64 |
| 246 | 111.82 | | |

## CHART 2
## AUTOMATIC CALCULATION FOR BODY SURFACE AREA

| Height in inches | Height in meters | Body Surface Area |
|---|---|---|
| 48 | 1.22 | 1.49 |
| 49 | 1.24 | 1.55 |
| 50 | 1.27 | 1.61 |
| 51 | 1.30 | 1.68 |
| 52 | 1.32 | 1.74 |
| 53 | 1.35 | 1.81 |
| 54 | 1.37 | 1.88 |
| 55 | 1.40 | 1.95 |
| 56 | 1.42 | 2.02 |
| 57 | 1.45 | 2.10 |
| 58 | 1.47 | 2.17 |
| 59 | 1.50 | 2.25 |
| 60 | 1.52 | 2.32 |
| 61 | 1.55 | 2.40 |
| 62 | 1.57 | 2.48 |
| 63 | 1.60 | 2.56 |
| 64 | 1.63 | 2.64 |
| 65 | 1.65 | 2.73 |
| 66 | 1.68 | 2.81 |
| 67 | 1.70 | 2.90 |

| Height in inches | Height in meters | Body Surface Area |
|---|---|---|
| 68 | 1.73 | 2.98 |
| 69 | 1.75 | 3.07 |
| 70 | 1.78 | 3.16 |
| 71 | 1.80 | 3.25 |
| 72 | 1.83 | 3.34 |
| 73 | 1.85 | 3.44 |
| 74 | 1.88 | 3.53 |
| 75 | 1.91 | 3.63 |
| 76 | 1.93 | 3.73 |
| 77 | 1.96 | 3.83 |
| 78 | 1.98 | 3.93 |
| 79 | 2.01 | 4.03 |
| 80 | 2.03 | 4.13 |
| 81 | 2.06 | 4.23 |
| 82 | 2.08 | 4.34 |
| 83 | 2.11 | 4.44 |
| 84 | 2.13 | 4.55 |

# **Notes**

**INTRODUCTION**

**1.** R. Sichieri, "Relative Weight Classifications in the Assessment of Underweight and Overweight in the United States," *International Journal of Obesity* 16, no. 4 (1992): 303–12.

**2.** Ibid.

**3.** National Center for Health Statistics, U.S. Department of Health and Human Services (1985).

**4.** K. Kohima et al., "The Association between Body Mass Index and Self-Assessed Symptoms among Young Women," *Nippon Koshu Eisei Zasshi* (*Japanese Journal of Public Health*) 41, no. 2 (1994): 126–30.

**5.** R. F. Kushner, "Body Weight and Mortality," *Nutrition Reviews* 51, no. 5 (1993): 127–36.

**6.** S. Cattanach, "Pregnancy Hazards Associated with Low Maternal Body Mass Indices," *Australian and New Zealand Journal of Obstetrics and Gynaecology* 33, no. 1 (1993): 45–47.

**7.** Ibid.


**AN OPEN LETTER TO MY FELLOW PHYSICIANS**

**1.** R. Sichieri, "Relative Weight Classifications in the Assessment of Underweight and Overweight in the United States," *International Journal of Obesity* 16, no. 4 (1992): 303–12.

**2.** National Center for Health Statistics, U.S. Department of Health and Human Services.

## 1 THE NEW WAY TO TELL IF YOU'RE UNDERWEIGHT

**1.** R. Sichieri, "Relative Weight Classifications in the Assessment of Underweight and Overweight in the United States," *International Journal of Obesity and Related Metabolic Disorders* 16, no. 4 (1992): 303–12; R. F. Kushner, "Body Weight and Mortality," *Nutrition Reviews* 51, no. 5 (1993): 127–36.

**2.** S. Cattanach, "Pregnancy Hazards Associated with Low Maternal Body Mass Indices," *Australian and New Zealand Journal of Obstetrics and Gynaecology* 33, no. 1 (1993): 45–47.

**3.** T. R. Knapp, "A Methodological Critique of the 'Ideal Weight' Concept," *Journal of the American Medical Association* 250 (1983): 506–10; G. G. Harrison, "Height-Weight Tables," *Annals of Internal Medicine* 100 (1984): 285–95.

**4.** Jerome M. Hershman and G. A. Bray, eds., *The Thyroid: Physiology and Treatment of Disease* (1978).

**5.** C. R. Kannan, *The Pituitary Gland* (1987).

## 2 WHAT THEY NEVER TOLD YOU ABOUT UNDERWEIGHT

**1.** Lund-Larsen et al., "Changes in Smoking Habits and Body Weight," *Journal of Chronic Diseases* 35 (1982): 773–80.

**2.** B. Spring et al., "Weight Gain and Withdrawal Symptoms after Smoking Cessation," *Health Psychology* (in press).

**3.** D. T. Dempsey, "Prognostic Value of Nutritional Indices," *Journal of Parenteral and Enteral Nutrition* 1, 5 Suppl. (1987): 109–45.

**4.** R. Sichieri, "Relative Weight Classifications in the Assessment of Underweight and Overweight in the United States," *International Journal of Obesity and Related Metabolic Disorders* 16, no. 4 (1992): 303–12.

**5.** "Diet, Nutrition, and the Prevention of Chronic Disease," *World Health Organization Technical Report* 797 (1990): 69–71.

**6.** R. S. Gibson, *Principles of Nutritional Assessment* (New York: Oxford University Press, 1990).

## 3 HOW TO GAIN WITH "FRIENDLY FAT"

**1.** L. Lapidus, "Distribution of Adipose Tissue and Risk of Cardiovascular Disease and Death," *British Medical Journal* 289 (1984): 1257–61.

**2.** "Human Nutrition," *Grolier Multimedia Encyclopedia* (1992).

**3.** "Diet, Nutrition, and the Prevention of Chronic Disease," *World Health Organization Technical Report* 797 (1990): 69–71.

**4.** A. P. Fitzgerald, "Body Weight and Coronary Heart Disease Mortality," *International Journal of Obesity* 16 (1992): 119–23.

**5.** D. V. Schapira, "Obesity, Body Fat Distribution, and Sex Hormones," *Cancer* 67 (1991): 2215–18.

#### 4 CARBOHYDRATES: PICK THEM RIGHT TO PUT ON POUNDS

**1.** Dr. David Reuben, *The Save-Your-Life Diet* (New York: Random House, 1975).

**2.** R. D. Guthrie, *Guthrie and Honeyman's Introduction to Carbohydrate Chemistry,* 4th ed. (1974).

**3.** W. Pigman, *Carbohydrates: Chemistry and Biochemistry,* 2d ed. (1980).

**4.** P. B. Foster, *Carbohydrate Chemistry* (1979).

**5.** D. T. Dempsey, "Prognostic Value of Nutritional Indices," *Journal of Parenteral and Enteral Nutrition* 1, 5 Suppl. (1987): 109–45.

**6.** William J. Kaufman, *Guide to Carbohydrates* (1978); John Kennedy, ed., *Carbohydrate Chemistry* (1988).

#### 5 WEIGHT GAIN STRATEGY: THE KEY TO SUCCESS

**1.** T. R. Knapp, "A Methodological Critique of the 'Ideal Weight' Concept," *Journal of the American Medical Association* 250 (1983): 506–10.

**2.** G. A. Bray, "Pathophysiology of Obesity," *American Journal of Clinical Nutrition* 55 (1992): 488S–94S.

**3.** D. V. Schapira, "Obesity, Body Fat Distribution, and Sex Hormones," *Cancer* 67 (1991): 2215–18.

**4.** J. E. Manson, "A Prospective Study of Obesity and Risk of Coronary Heart Disease in Women," *New England Journal of Medicine* 322 (1990); 88209.

**5.** B. Larson, "Is Abdominal Body Fat Distribution a Major Explanation of the Sex Difference in the Incidence of Myocardial Infarction?" *American Journal of Epidemiology* 135 (1992): 266–73.

#### 6 THE CALORIC BILL OF RIGHTS, CCK, OFD, AND OTHER TRICKS OF THE TRADE

**1.** C. T. Dourish, "Postponement of Satiety by Blockade of Brain CCK Receptors," *Science* 245 (1989): 1509–14.

**2.** G. F. Smith, "Are Gut Peptides a New Class of Anorectic Agents?" *American Journal of Clinical Nutrition* (1992): 55.

**3.** J. F. Morley, "The Neuroendocrine Control of Appetite; the Role of the Endogenous Opiates, Cholecystokinin, etc.," *Life Sciences* 27, no. 5 (1980): 355–68.

**4.** E. Phillip, "Disturbed Cholecystokinin Secretion in Patients with Eating Disorders," *Life Sciences* 48 (1991): 2443–50.

**5.** B. Beck, "Cholecystokinin, Neurotensin, and Corticotropin-Releasing Factor, etc.," *Annales D'Endocrinologie (Paris)* 53, no. 1 (1992): 44–56.

**6.** S. Holt, "Relationship of Satiety to Postprandial Glycaemic, Insulin and Cholecystokinin Responses," *Appetite* 18, no. 2 (1992): 129–42.

**7.** R. A. Liddle, "Cholecystokinin Bioactivity in Human Plasma, etc.," *Journal of Clinical Investigation* 75 (1985): 1144–52.

### 7 PUTTING THE PROGRAM TO WORK FOR YOU: MORE CALORIES WITH EVERY BITE

**1.** E. F. Hinsch, "The Role of Lipids in Atherosclerosis," *Physiology Reviews* 23 (1943): 185.

**2.** S. L. Malhotra, "Serum Lipids Dietary Factors and Ischemic Heart Disease," *American Journal of Clinical Nutrition* 20 (1967): 462.

**3.** R. G. Gould, "Lipid Metabolism and Atherosclerosis," *Journal of the American Medical Association* 11 (1951): 209.

**4.** Dr. David R. Reuben, *Everything You Always Wanted to Know about Nutrition* (New York: Avon, 1979), 111.

### 10 HOW VEGETARIANS CAN GAIN WEIGHT EASILY: THE ORGANOLEPTIC CONNECTION

**1.** Dr. David Reuben, *The Save-Your-Life Diet* (New York: Random House, 1975); Dr. David Reuben, *The Save-Your-Life Diet High Fiber Cook Book* (New York: Random House, 1976).

### 12 SENIORS CAN DO IT TOO: WHEN MORE POUNDS MEAN LONGER LIFE

**1.** J. F. Morley, "The Neuroendocrine Control of Appetite; the Role of the Endogenous Opiates, Cholecystokinin, etc.," *Life Sciences* 27, no. 5 (1980): 355–68.

**2.** Ibid.

### 15 MORE FUN: EASY HI-CAL RECIPES YOU CAN MAKE IN A JIFFY

**1.** Dr. David Reuben, *The Save-Your-Life Diet* (New York: Random House, 1975).

# Index